Table of Con

Intermittent fasting for women

Fat burning on the stomach & low carb recipes
Lose weight on the stomach Incl. 31 exercises &
55 recipes - the best of 3 worlds 3in1
Author: Emma katie

Contents

Introduction

There's a reason intermittent fasting is one of the most popular diets in the world today: it works! More specifically, it helps people not only lose the weight they want (which you will learn in the book), but also get and stay healthy. While it's not a magic pill to make all your adipose tissues and diseases go away, it can help you reach your ideal weight and greatly reduce your risk of certain health problems. In this book, I'm going to show you what intermittent fasting really is, why you should incorporate it into your lifestyle, how it can help you stay slim and healthy, the different types of intermittent fasting (protocols), and how to do intermittent fasting Fasting as a lifestyle lives with a list of things you should and shouldn't do. By the time you finish reading this book, you will be able to incorporate intermittent fasting into your lifestyle and on your way to becoming leaner and healthier.

Chapter 1: Intermittent Basics of Fasting

To understand what intermittent fasting is and why you can benefit from it, it is important to break the term down into its constituent parts - fasting and intermittent. First, let's talk about fasting. There are many different impressions of the word "fasting". For some people, it's a diet. For some, it is a way of twisting God's arm to get what they want from him - as if they could twist God's arm. For some, it is a way of purifying the body.

So what is fasting really? Basically, fasting is the act of deliberately staying away from food for a period of time. When fasting, you either eat no food at all or only very little. Most people know fasting as an act of gaining God's favor, such as B. in Islam. In these and other religions, fasting is one of the best ways to "please" God (be it with the intention of simply pleasing him or obtaining his blessings), to pay for the sins they have committed or to give their spirits to strengthen and become more sensitive to God's voice.

The latter perception of spiritual strengthening and tightening is surprisingly supported by psychological principles, albeit from a different point of view. How is that meant? For people who are very religious or devout, the ability to withstand the temptations of the world such as sex, vice and materialism, among others, depends on the strength of one's mind. There is a very good spiritual analogy that illustrates the struggle between the spirit and the flesh, or worldly desires - the good and bad inner wolves.

The Native American Indians believe that there are 2 wolves living within a person's mind, both of whom are at odds with one another. The stronger wolf is the one who makes the person think, feel and live their life in a certain way, that is, good or bad. And who determines who is stronger between the two wolves? The person himself. When a person starves his carnal wolf, the bad one, he weakens it and inadvertently feeds the good wolf to make it strong, and vice versa. Fasting is one of the main ways in which most religions feed the good wolf and, consequently, starve the bad one.

That is why religious people believe that fasting strengthens the spirit, that is, the good wolf, to fight temptation. In the field of psychology, the term relating to the practice of starving the bad wolf refers to delayed gratification. If you remember what happened to children in the famous marshmallow test, those who were able to resist the excitement of eating the marshmallows immediately grew into well-adjusted and disciplined adults. Because fasting involves a lot of delayed gratification, it allows a person to develop a much stronger character or willpower. Why starve?

Believe it or not, the benefits of fasting aren't just limited to the mind or psyche. It extends to the physical body as well. Well, how can starving for an extended period of time have health benefits when folk science claims that starving for an extended period of time is no good. Isn't food one of the essential requirements for longevity? While it is true that food is a prerequisite for staying alive and hunger is generally not good for the body and mind, conscious starvation for a limited amount of time is actually much healthier, both physically and mentally.

The key to this is rapid or periodic fasting. That brings us to the second word of the term, which is "intermittent". To get the benefits of fasting and the desired health effects, it is important to fast intermittently and not for long periods of time, such as when you are fasting. B. for days or weeks. Here are the top health benefits of intermittent fasting:

Accelerated fat loss

Losing weight isn't necessarily a great thing, especially when you're losing the wrong weight. "Really?" Is There a Right Type of Weight Loss? Yes, there is and it's called fat loss! Many people confuse weight loss with fat loss, which is why so many unhealthy quick weight loss diets - aka crash diets - continue to be so prevalent on the internet and beyond. While it is true that many crash diets can really make a person lose 5 pounds or more a week, it is worth noting that most of the weight lost is of the type that one does not want to lose:

Water and muscle mass. Intermittent fasting helps you lose the right type of weight at a fast but healthy pace - body fat. Believe me, even if you lose less than 1 kilo per week (the established healthy weight loss rate), 4 pounds of body fat in a month (at 4 weeks per month), you will look significantly leaner compared to 8 pounds in a month because that loss is mostly water and muscle.

Why the need to maintain as much muscle mass as possible? The more muscle you have, the faster your metabolism is.

This one has the ability to burn calories and stored body fat. If you lose mostly body fat and minimal muscle mass, your metabolism will hardly change and you will mostly burn body fat! Intermittent fasting speeds up your metabolism by increasing the production of fat-burning hormones like norepinephrine while minimizing insulin production. Studies have shown that, on average, intermittent fasting - if done correctly - can help your body burn up to 14% more calories and body fat.

In particular, a 2014 review of a certain section of the scientific literature showed that intermittent fasting can help people lose up to 8% of their weight within 24 weeks, which can be considered significant weight loss for a relatively short period of time. Imagine if you weigh 100 pounds you can lose up to 8 pounds in just 6 months or less! The same study also found that those who participated in the study lost up to 7% of their waistlines.

This shows that the greatest weight loss that was achieved was body fat. Another study showed that intermittent fasting retained more muscle mass compared to low-calorie diets. The reason? Remember how intermittent fasting increases the production of fat burning hormones while minimizing fat storing hormones? Now you know why. Because of its ability to increase your calorie consumption and improve your metabolism, intermittent fasting can help you achieve your weight loss, body fat loss, and goals.

Minimizing type 2 diabetes

One of the most common health epidemics in the world is diabetes. In many countries around the world, particularly affluent countries or the First World, diabetes is becoming one of the deadliest diseases that governments have to contend with. This medical condition is primarily the result of increased insulin resistance (low insulin sensitivity), which makes a person's blood sugar levels consistently high and chronic. Conversely, the lower a person's insulin resistance (high sensitivity), the lower their blood sugar is usually.

As mentioned earlier, intermittent fasting can help minimize the production of insulin. Several studies have estimated that intermittent fasting can lower insulin levels by up to 31%.
In this context, it has also been estimated, based on studies, that intermittent fasting can help lower blood sugar levels by up to 6%. By improving insulin sensitivity (reducing insulin resistance) and lowering blood sugar levels, intermittent fasting can help minimize the risk of developing type 2 diabetes.

However, this benefit is more applicable to men than women. One study showed that women's blood sugar levels rose on average during a 3-week intermittent fasting protocol.

Improved Cardiovascular Health

Today ISIS or the Syrian army are not the greatest murderers in the world. They are cardiovascular diseases. And there are health markers or risk factors that can help determine your risk of heart disease. One of the benefits of intermittent fasting is reducing some of these markers or risk factors, which include high cholesterol, high blood pressure, blood sugar levels, triglyceride levels, and markers of inflammation. I say "likely" because these benefits have mainly been seen in animals, which means more studies - in humans - need to be done on the cardiovascular benefits of intermittent fasting.

That said, the likelihood that such benefits would also apply to humans is high, considering that most scientific tests for the possible effects of drugs and other things are tested on animals first. And often the positive test results give the researchers and scientists the signal to apply such things on humans.

Improved cellular recovery

One process that is critical to cell repair is the removal of waste from the cells, that is. Autophagy. This includes the metabolism of dysfunctional or broken proteins that can build up in cells over time.

Increased autophagy can help metabolize or remove more of such broken or dysfunctional proteins and, consequently, improve the body's cellular repair function. Intermittent fasting can help your body achieve increased autophagy and in the process help your body repair cells much better.

Cellular gene and hormonal changes

If you haven't eaten in a long time, several important hormonal changes happen. As already mentioned, this includes an increased production of the fat-burning hormone norepinephrine and a lowering of the insulin level. As mentioned earlier, it also includes increased autophagy, which leads to better cell repair.

Another hormonal change that can occur intermittently during fasting is increased production of human growth hormones, which can help you gain more muscle or even maintain muscle mass while dieting. Besides looking a lot fitter, having more muscle will help you get stronger.

Reduced levels of oxidative stress and inflammation

The most common cause of premature aging and most chronic and degenerative diseases today is oxidative stress. Why? Because it hits your body where it matters most - at the cellular level! Oxidative stress involves the reaction of free radicals or unstable molecules to the body's crucial molecules such as protein and DNA. And such reactions are not good - they are harmful and dangerous!

Scientific studies have shown that intermittent fasting has the beneficial ability to help the body strengthen its ability to fight off or fight off oxidative stress. Some studies have also shown that intermittent fasting can also reduce another major factor in many chronic diseases: **inflammation.** Hence, intermittent fasting is one of the best ways to slow aging and reduce the risks for many of today's chronic and degenerative diseases.

Better management of cancer

Some studies, albeit done on animals, have shown that intermittent fasting can help reduce risks of certain types of cancer through improved metabolic processes. In human studies, intermittent fasting has been shown to help minimize the side effects of chemotherapy.

Optimal mind

Often times, what is good for the body in general is also good for the brain. Better metabolism, substantial improvements in insulin and blood sugar le
vels, reduction of oxidative stress and reduced inflammation can all contribute to optimal cognitive and mental performance as well as general brain health. Animal studies have shown that

intermittent fasting can help grow new nerve cells, which are critical to optimal mental performance and brain health.

According to a study, while fasting, it stimulates the production of brain-derived neurotropic factor (BDNF), an important hormone that can help reduce risks for mental health problems such as depression, among others. Finally, intermittent fasting can also help minimize the harmful effects of stroke on the brain.

Lower risk of Alzheimer's disease

One of the most common neurodegenerative diseases in the world is Alzheimer's disease. At present there is still no known cure for Alzheimer's disease, despite scientific breakthroughs that bring us closer to the discovery of such a remedy. At this point, the best medicine is still prevention. While studies that have shown significant insight into the role of intermittent fasting in lowering the risk of Alzheimer's have been conducted in animals, that does not mean that intermittent fasting does not mean that the anti-Alzheimer's benefits are not applicable to humans. Keep in mind that most of the scientific breakthroughs in the medical field were first validated in animals before they were validated in humans. Therefore, intermittent fasting may help reduce your risk of Alzheimer's and even Parkinson's and Huntington's. And while there are no significant studies of people to date that confirm the role of intermittent fasting in the fight against Alzheimer's, there are reports that Alzheimer's patients have much better symptoms after fasting for a short period of time as an intervention method.

Generally longer life

Eventually, general improvements in general health will improve life expectancy. Since intermittent fasting can help achieve the important health and fitness benefits noted above, it is very likely that including intermittent fasting as part of a generally healthy lifestyle can help extend life.

In the next few chapters, we'll look at the most popular ways intermittent fasting is performed around the world, commonly referred to as protocols. Each protocol has its own unique benefits that can help you incorporate temporary fasting into your lifestyle, regardless of your personal circumstances.

Chapter 2: The Lean Gain Protocol

This is considered to be one of the most popular rapid fasting protocols in the world. The proponent of this protocol is Martin Berkhan. The Lean Gains Protocol is ideal for you if you like to lift the weights in the gym and want to be defined, i.e. build muscle and lose body fat.

How it works

If you are a man you have to fast 16 hours every day and if you are a woman you have to fast for a shorter time every day - 14 hours.

The remaining 8 (men) to 10 (women) hours will be your feeding or eating window. You will not go completely without food during your 14 to 16 hour daily fast. During this time you can still eat something, but only calorie-free. Drinking (preferably water or other calorie-free drinks) is also allowed. At the top of the list, of course, is water! Other acceptable alternatives include calorie-free sodas and chewing gum, unsweetened black coffee (or sweetened with a calorie-free sweetener such as stevia), and tea. When should you start fasting and for how long? It depends on you, but the best time would be when you are the least likely to find yourself fasting. For most people, their ideal fasting time is during the night - it's easier to fast while you sleep - until late in the morning. For such people, late morning is usually 6 hours after waking up.

If you are the type of person who is very hectic most of the time, the timing of your meal window can be such as to suit the most stressful or hectic times of your days and provide you with the energy you need when you are at it most need. And if you plan your Lent during your quietest times, you can be flexible. Aside from the times when you can and are not allowed to eat, watch out for what you can and cannot eat.

In particular, you need to consider the types of foods that are optimal for your regular gym workouts. The days you go to the gym, you need more carbohydrates for fuel and fewer fat calories. But on non-gym days, more fat calories than carbohydrates are better. Why? Fat calories are more filling, therefore filling, which can help keep you feeling full longer and reduce your cravings or hunger levels during your fasting window. But whether or not you hit the gym, you need to make sure you are providing adequate protein for muscle loss or for building muscle.

Regardless of the type of calories you eat, it is important to eat whole and unprocessed foods. Every now and then, there aren't any downsides to processed items like a replacement shake or granola bar, especially if you're looking for a quick fix. Just make sure that eating processed foods is the exception rather than the norm.

As with all good things, this protocol has its own advantages and disadvantages. First, let's talk about the benefit of being that there will be no fuss about meal frequency.

Eating all in one meal or 20 meals doesn't matter as long as you only eat in your designated eating window. For many people, being able to choose how often they are allowed to eat on a given day is a great blessing that allows them to practice intermittent fasting.

Chapter 3: The Eat-Stop-Eat Protocol

This intermittent fasting protocol was created by a man named Brad Pilon. If you are the type of person who already eats properly and healthily then this might be the protocol for you. Compared to some of the relatively extreme diet protocols, the Eat-Stop-Eat protocol was mostly geared towards moderation. What do i mean by that? You can eat pretty much anything you like here, as long as you only eat moderate amounts of it. So, if you want to have a slice of pizza, go for it! Just make sure it only sticks to one piece and you don't eat the rest.

How it works

With the Eat-Stop-Eat method, you don't have to fast every day. You have to do it no more than twice a week for 24 hours each time. And during these 24 hour fasts you are not allowed to eat anything, but you can freely drink any drink as long as it has no calories, e.g. B. Water and green tea. When your fast is over, just return to your usual eating routine. You also have the freedom to choose the timing of your weekly fast.

This means that you can schedule your fasts or fasts on days when you have the least difficulty in fasting for 24 hours. For some people, it's the weekends, while for others, it's the busiest days that they barely notice when they are hungry. It's really up to you. As mentioned earlier, this protocol is all about moderation. As such, it aims to reduce your calorie consumption by reducing your meal frequency for the whole week, e.g. B. Not to eat 1 or 2 days a week. By doing this, you inadvertently cut down on your weekly calorie intake on the way to losing fat.

Regular exercise is another important part of this protocol. Weight lifting or weight training is the best thing you can do. Why? By exercising, you minimize muscle loss and increase fat loss. And as I mentioned earlier, one of the most important factors in determining how much calories your body can burn on a regular basis and how much body fat you can lose while dieting is one of the most important factors I mentioned.

Advantages and disadvantages

When it comes to the eat-stop-eat protocol, its greatest asset is flexibility. Why? This is because you can start small with this protocol and take small, but then larger, steps towards full implementation. You can fast for as long as possible during the first or second day and gradually increase the duration of your fast as your body responds accordingly. Brad Pilon - the creator and main proponent of the protocol - advocates that you follow the protocol on what may be the most active day of your week or on a day when you don't have to make social commitments (minimizing the temptation to eat). If you start the protocol on a day marked by at least one of the two conditions, you may be able to focus your mind too much on being aware of the food (or its lack of it) to minimize the temptation to fast your early to break, or both. Another important benefit of the protocol is that there are no prohibited foods or an obligation to monitor your calories.

The fact that you don't have to closely monitor what and how much you eat makes this protocol much less difficult to implement compared to many other intermittent fasting methods. Still, it's important to remember that this protocol isn't a free ticket to swallow every day like it's the end of the world. The key - as with everything else - is moderation. Eat anything you want, but remember not to overdo it. As for the cons, the only one associated with the Eat-Stop-Eat protocol is the duration of fasting, which is at least 24 hours. Without food once or twice a week for 24 hours can still be challenging for most people, especially during the first few weeks of following the protocol when side effects can occur. This may include irritability, headache, fatigue, or anxiety, which will gradually go away after the first few weeks. If you choose to implement this protocol, you should know that 24-hour fasting is very demanding, even if you slowly increase your fasting period. Therefore, the temptation to eat every time you break your fast can be very strong. This is where you need to stay strong and make sure you eat moderately when breaking your fast under this protocol.

Chapter 4: The Protocol of the Warrior Diet

As the name suggests, this protocol requires you to eat like a "warrior". And what does it mean to eat like a warrior? The author of the protocol, Ori Hofmekler, believes that ancient warriors only ate one large meal a day, namely dinner. For the remainder of the 24 hours, these warriors fasted.

How it works

This type of diet is explained very simply - eat one large meal each day and one in the evening. That's it. Very easy, isn't it? But why should you plan your big meal in the evening, which is contrary to what many conventional nutritionists say? Because according to Hofmekler, humans are night eaters due to their genetic make-up. Given this particular genetic predisposition, it only makes sense to plan your one large meal in the evening so that you can optimally supply your body with all the nutrients it needs. Hofmekler explains that this is because the parasympathetic nervous system is able to help the body relax, digest food, recover and calm down, which is conducive to maximum cell repair and growth.

Additionally, Hofmekler claims that eating just one large meal in the evening can also help produce important hormones and consequently burn more body fat during the day. And when you do this you also need to consider the order in which you will eat certain types of foods during your 4 hour meal window.

He recommends that you eat your vegetables first, proteins next, and fats last. And if you're still hungry despite your one big meal, you can eat more carbohydrates.

From the perspective of the Warrior Diet Protocol, fasting is about starving below average. This can help you increase your energy levels, optimize fat burning, and increase mental alertness during fasting by increasing or strengthening the flight or fight response of your sympathetic nervous system.

Advantages and disadvantages

The main benefit of the Warrior Diet Protocol is that it is technically not burdensome as it allows you to eat small portions of raw vegetables, fruits, proteins, and juices during your daily 20-hour fast. This can make it a lot easier for you to implement it consistently and stick with it for the long term. Others reported significant improvements in energy levels and the ability to burn body fat.

Since you are limited to vegetables, lean protein, and good dietary fat, and you can only eat in the evenings, it can be difficult to attend most social events while strictly following protocol. Another potential downside, especially early on, is the difficulty of eating almost all of your daily evening caloric needs in one meal. This can be more pronounced considering that most people are used to eating most of their daily nutritional needs during the day. But over time this can become less of a challenge as you gradually get used to the evening meal.

Chapter 5: The Alternate Day Protocol

This protocol was prepared by Dr. James Johnson created. Compared to the other intermittent fasting protocols, the Alternate Day Diet can be considered one of the simpler protocols to implement.

With this protocol, you fast every other day. E.g. you eat very little on your fasting days and normal the days in between.

How it works

But what does eating very little mean? Because we have to be honest, the term means different things to different people.

For a Shaquille O'Neal who is 7 feet 1 inches tall and weighs 324 pounds, the term "very little" can already be considered a buffet for Isaiah Thomas, who stands only 5 feet 9 inches and weighs just over 185 pounds. For the purposes of this protocol, "very little" means getting only 20% of your daily caloric needs or expenditure.

So if you typically consume 2,500 calories a day, you are only consuming 500 calories on your fasting days. For the sake of simplicity, Dr. Johnson recommends drinking meal replacement shakes on the days you are fasting. Such shakes are easy to consume throughout the day and they can contain a lot of nutrients. But dr. Johnson recommends not making a habit. He says that after the first two weeks after starting the protocol, you should return to eating real whole foods during your fast.

And remember, like we mentioned about regular weight lifting as part of the Warrior Diet Protocol. Weight lifting is also an important part of the Alternate Day protocol.

Because of this, the best time to plan your exercise is on the days when you are not fasting. This will help you get the most out of your workouts and get the most of them.

Advantages and disadvantages

The Alternate Day Protocol is one that is primarily designed to help you lose the healthy type of weight, body fat. When you lose more body fat than water or muscle mass in terms of weight, you will not only look fit but also feel fit.

You will also be much healthier. Based on Dr. Johnson's website allows you to lose up to a pound a week, which is considered a safe weight loss pace by most health and fitness experts.

Another advantage of this protocol is its relative simplicity. No need to count calories or watch what you eat. It's one less burden on your mind. But its relative simplicity can also be a disadvantage in reducing your calories to just 20% of your usual caloric needs every other day, which can be too much if you are not used to fasting. While it can be easy not to eat all day practically every day, for some it is not the easiest thing in the world. There is also a higher risk of binge eating on normal days.

Chapter 6: The Fat Loss Forever Protocol

This intermittent fasting protocol was developed by Dan Go and John Romaniello. This protocol combines the best of the Lean Gains, Eat-Stop-Eat and Warrior Diet protocols into one. Think of it as a 3-in-1 pack of coffee, only that it's intermittent fasting. Two of its main characteristics are a push-and-pull relationship, or heaven and hell. One day a week you can have cheat meals (heaven) followed by a 36 hour fast (hell).

The other 5 days will then be split between the 3 different protocols according to your wishes. The creator of the protocol suggests that you plan your longest fast on the days when you are most active. Why? So your mind is too busy to ponder or notice hunger brewing in your stomach. You can purchase the plan of the protocol from Dan and John's website and get free exercise programs (body weight and free weight exercises) that can help you get the most out of your healthy weight loss (fat loss) efforts.

Advantages and disadvantages

Its main pro is that the 7-day fasting cycle lets your body get used to fasting and thus gives it structure. As a result, you can maximize the fat burning and muscle building results of the protocol and your exercise program. With the Fat-Loss-Forever-Protocol you can fast in a structured, controlled and effective way. Its disadvantage? Well, similar to other protocols, after the longest fast of the week, 36 hours, the temptation to binge eat is very high compared to the other protocols because you fast longer.

Another potential downside to the protocol - at least at first glance - is that it can be very confusing or difficult to strictly follow. Why? It is because of its strict but very different schedules during the 7 day cycle. Remember that for five days you will be doing the three protocols mentioned above that will prevent you from establishing a rhythm or pattern. But if you continue with the protocol like this, you will eventually get used to it.

Chapter 7: The 5: 2 Diet Protocol

The 5: 2 protocol, also known as the Fast Diet, is one of the most popular, if not the most popular, of the intermittent fasting protocols these days.

How it works

This protocol from British journalist and Doctor Michael Mosley fasts 2 days a week and not the other 5 days. Now you might be wondering, isn't that exactly how the eat-stop-eat method works? On the surface, it seems that way. But actually that's not the case. For one, you can fast only one day during the week using the Eat-Stop-Eat protocol, while you can fast for two days using the 5: 2 protocol. Another important difference is that you can eat under the 5: 2 protocol during the 2 days of fasting, while with the Eat-Stop-Eat method you are only allowed to enjoy calorie-free drinks during the fast. When talking about calories, a woman is allowed to consume a total of 500 calories and 600 calories if you are a man. There are no "rules", you can eat what you want and when you want.

For example:

● Three (3) mini meals, one each at breakfast, lunch and dinner,

or

● Two (2) smaller meals, usually with lunch and dinner. Remember, the only rule here is to limit your calorie intake to a maximum of 600 and 500 calories on the fasting days if you are a man or a woman. Therefore, you should distribute your calories sensibly throughout the day. While there are no "right" or "wrong" foods under this protocol, there are wise and unwise choices.

Foods high in fiber and protein tend to be wise choices as they can help you feel full longer and can significantly reduce hunger pangs. In turn, these can help you keep your calories within the daily limit.

Another wise food choice are soups that are made from whole food ingredients.

This does not mean instant soups. They are not good for your health or your waistline. The only other rule to follow as part of this protocol is to make sure that there is at least 1 normal day of eating in between your 2 days of fasting.

Many people who follow this protocol schedule their fast every Monday and Thursday, eat 3 small meals on each of those days, and then eat normally for the remaining days. Speaking of normal food, please don't confuse it with "eat as much as you can". Eat the same amount as you normally would if you weren't fasting.

Advantages and disadvantages

One of the advantages of this protocol is that it doesn't really feel like a diet because it is more of an eating pattern than a "diet." Not only do you get small portions to eat on the fasting days, but it is only 2 days a week, you also have no restrictions on the type of food. Therefore, it is easier for many people to follow this protocol than most other intermittent fasting protocols or weight loss diets. The only downside to this protocol from my point of view is that you won't lose as much weight as you would with the other protocols because it is milder in terms of calorie consumption. Your fasting days are more likely to be "severe calorie restriction" days than days without food. But if you think you aren't ambitious enough to lose more weight on the other tougher protocols, it's fine. Each to their own, and if this protocol suits you best, then be sure to go into it.

Chapter 8: The Spontaneous Fasting Protocol

The last protocol we'll look at is what I would consider Intermittent Fasting Lite because it's the simplest of all protocols.

How it works

As the name suggests, there are no rules as to when you will fast.

Fasting under this protocol is much like watching movies on Netflix. Here you do not have to adhere to a specific structure in order to be able to fast temporarily. Just skip meals every now and then, especially if you are not yet hungry or are so busy that you cannot afford to eat. Just make sure you are eating nutritious and healthy meals when you decide to eat. In short, the spontaneous fasting protocol is a more organic method of intermittent fasting by skipping a meal or two a day when it suits you.

Advantages and disadvantages

Obviously, the biggest benefit here is the lack of structure. You can skip your meals at the most convenient times of the day and there are no prohibited foods. So there is really no reason you couldn't fast intermittently except for one thing: you don't really want to do it. But its greatest advantage can also be its greatest disadvantage. Some people need structure to get things done, and if you are such a person, the lack of structure in this diet can make it difficult for you to implement it successfully.

Another downside to this intermittent fasting protocol is that it is easiest when it is easiest, it can produce the slightest positive results, especially when it comes to healthy weight loss. Healthy weight loss always works through a reduction in calories and in a consistent state of a calorie deficit, ie taking in fewer calories than are consumed or burned.

A protocol that is not based on a consistent effort to significantly reduce calories is one that will save you from optimal weight or fat loss. Either you lose significantly more weight than the other protocols, or you lose significantly less weight over a period of time compared to the other protocols. This is the tradeoff between expediency and results.

Chapter 9: Muscles - The Secret to Getting and Staying Lean

When it comes to healthy weight loss (body fat), diet or diet is only part of the equation. Another important consideration -

perhaps even more important - is your metabolism, or the rate at which your body can burn calories or body fat. The higher your metabolism, the more calories or body fat your body can burn. A faster metabolism coupled with a reduction in calories is a potent double punch against body fat. And when it comes to metabolism, one of the most important factors that affect it is the amount of muscle mass your body has.

Why is that? Of all the cells in your body, muscles are the most metabolically active and require the most calories for normal function.

It follows that the more muscle you have, the faster your metabolism can be and, consequently, when your muscle mass is reduced, your metabolism slows down. When it comes to maintaining or even increasing muscle mass while fasting, there are many "passionate" discussions.

Many who take the conventional point of view say that a severe caloric restriction - as is the case with fasting - leads to muscle breakdown and therefore muscle breakdown. But how true are statements like this? To answer this question, we need to consider two things. First, the types of calories you are consuming. The second is the timing of consumption. The following handy tips will help you manage these two factors so that you can maintain or even increase muscle mass even while fasting.

Breakfast

Whether as a means to break your fast or a way to start it, aim to have something to eat in the morning according to your chosen fasting schedule. If you choose to fast at night, then break your day fast with - sorry the pun - a small breakfast to start your day on an energetic note. If you decide to fast during the day, do the same, that is, eat a small breakfast just before your fasting period to start the day a little more energized.

But considering that you want to get optimal metabolism through muscle mass, building or maintaining muscle mass must be your main focus or priority. And whether you choose to fast during the day or all night, a great way to keep your muscles well-fed and prepared for growth or maintenance is to have something to eat as soon as you wake up.

So what's the best morning meal for optimal muscle maintenance or growth? Eat as much as you can, using proteins that are slow to digest like cheese, red meat, and eggs. Why? Not only will you feel satiated longer, but you are supplying your muscles with the most important building block for growth or maintenance - protein. And aside from protein, you will also benefit from consuming carbohydrates as it can support your mental and physical performance throughout the day. When it comes to timing your fasting season, there is only one significant difference and that is the ability to spread your calorie consumption out.

When you fast in the evening, you can spread your calories all over your eating window because you are awake. If you choose to fast during the day, you can only eat your total calories in one large meal in the evening for the 24 hour period. Unless you want to wake up in the middle of the night to spread your daily calorie consumption over several meals.

Schedule your workouts later in the day

Before lifting the weights or doing bodyweight exercises such as plyometrics or calisthenics, it is of the utmost importance that you are able to consume a significant amount of calories in order to do your exercises well and not pass out from exhaustion. And then later in the day when you go to the gym or do calisthenics or plyometrics, you can do that regardless of whether you go for the day or the night. If you are fasting during the day that ends late in the afternoon or early in the evening, say 6 p.m., it will do you good to plan your workouts later in the evening after you have had a chance to eat.

Aside from getting enough energy, exercising later in the evening increases your chances of getting the machines you feel like doing because most people are through with their workouts and you have less competition for the fitness equipment.

If you are fasting at night, it is best to exercise late in the afternoon or early in the evening.

So if you fast at 5 or 6 p.m., your best time to exercise is at 4 p.m. or 5 p.m., respectively. This gives you the opportunity to take your final calories before and immediately after your workout just before your fasting period begins. Can you imagine why you shouldn't exercise in the middle of the day?

It's not a good idea, especially if you are fasting during the day, because you won't be able to get enough calories for a meaningful exercise. If you work out in the morning it will be too much of a chore, especially if you have a day job.

Eat after exercise

Finally, you should do your best to plan for consuming the majority of your daily calories immediately after your workout. Why?
It is because of what is known as the 2-hour golden post-workout window, or also known as the anabolic window, in which your body's ability to recover and build muscle can be maximized through immediate post-workout nutrients.

And more importantly, the body's chances of storing all those extra calories from post-workout meals are lowest in that golden window because your body, especially your muscles, has all of the protein to rebuild and all of the carbohydrates, that it can get is needed to replenish its glycogen stores quickly, so is the primary fuel. And overeating before you work out will increase your chances of feeling lethargic and sluggish during your workout.

Chapter 10: Practical Tips for Intermittent Fasting Success

Make no mistake about it, intermittent fasting is one of the most effective ways to get in the best shape of your life and improve your health. However, it's not something that works for everyone.

Not a one-size-works-for-all thing. For some people, intermittent fasting can even be harmful to their health if they have pre-existing chronic illnesses, medical problems, or special dietary needs. If you are one of them, the first thing to do is to consult your doctor to see if intermittent fasting isn't going to be harmful to you if you suffer from your health condition or special dietary needs.

Assuming that you are generally healthy and have no particular nutritional needs, you must be very sensitive to the signals your body can give if you choose to fast intermittently.

You need to be able to sense when your body is doing well, calling for help and getting adequate medical attention, or when it is complaining about how uncomfortable intermittent fasting is for the first few weeks. Most people do not consider intermittent fasting "normal" and therefore it will really take some time to adjust to the lifestyle. And for women, fluctuating hormone levels can make it more difficult to start and stay on an intermittent fasting protocol than it is for men. When it comes to intermittent fasting, you should be more careful by being careful in the beginning and gradually moving from short fasts to much longer periods.

If, despite your best efforts and a few weeks in the lifestyle, you are still feeling extremely uncomfortable, there is no shame in accepting that intermittent fasting is not for you and that other dietary approaches may be your thing. To maximize your chances of making a successful transition to the intermittent fasting lifestyle, consider the following practical tips for starting your lifestyle.

Water

While you are in a phase of fasting, one of the most important - if not the most important - is the water you need. Unfortunately, many people who are in the intermittent fasting lifestyle are frequently dehydrated. And it's bad for you if you get dehydrated frequently during an intermittent fasting protocol. Why? Your body is mostly made up of water. Yes, up to 70% of your body is made up of that stuff, and as such, substantial drops in your body fluids can have subtle but substantial effects on your cells and nerves that can hinder optimal mental and physical performance.

Chronic dehydration can also make you prone to dizziness, constipation, dry skin, and fatigue, among others. And when you are fasting, drink pure water for hydration because everything else can contain high amounts of sugar and hidden calories, even if the labels say "sugar-free" or "zero calories". Another reason why you need to drink enough water while fasting for healthy weight loss, regardless of your chosen protocol, is because it helps you feel full longer.

This is why it is important to still drink a glass or two of water during the night, especially when you are fasting. It will help you minimize hunger pains. How much water is enough water? It is best to drink more than 8 glasses a day as you are fasting intermittently and, more importantly, when you exercise regularly. And make sure you have your water in multiple drinks throughout the day and night rather than just one or two drinks. Believe me, drinking your daily water needs in just one or two servings can be very uncomfortable if you do it regularly. While drinking very cold water is very refreshing, especially on hot days or nights, it is better if you drink room temperature or slightly cold water.

Why? Because very cold water can cause your blood vessels to contract and cause indigestion. The foods you eat in your eating window can also affect your hydration levels. One of the foods that you should minimize or avoid entirely is spicy because they tend to make you thirstier.

Salt is an ingredient that can make you significantly more thirsty than usual, so keep your consumption of very salty foods to a minimum. And if you eat very salty foods, be sure to increase your water intake to decrease the relatively strong taste. You can increase your chances of getting adequate hydration by eating fruits and vegetables that are fibrous and loaded with water. Aside from that, it also helps you feel full longer.

And if you want to enjoy a glass or two of fruit juices, don't go for commercially available ones, no matter how many manufacturers claim they are "all natural". The truth is, commercially available fruit juices are loaded with sugar, so the best way to drink freshly squeezed fruit juice is. This way, you can be 100% sure that what you are drinking does not contain excessive sugar or other harmful ingredients.

Plan your Lent

The timing of your fasts can be an important factor in making intermittent fasting long enough to experience its benefits. This can be even more crucial if you want to maximize fat loss from regular gym workouts. Most people who fast have day jobs and other large tasks to attend to.

Therefore, choosing the optimal time for your fasting phases is of central importance for you. This is why most people tend to plan their fasts throughout the evening and into the morning. This enables them to eat when they need it most, namely during the day when energy consumption is lowest. So if you are seriously considering diving into the intermittent fasting lifestyle, consider determining your evening fast, where the risk of breaking your fast prematurely is lowest.

Strength training

You should definitely lift weights if you really want to burn body fat, it will keep you looking healthy and fit. This is why I recommend weight lifting or resistance exercises, including calisthenics and plyometrics, as the primary form of regular exercise. And again, the reason is that resistance exercises or weight lifting are best for both burning fat and building muscle. I've seen friends who just lost weight without exercising and when they lost weight they looked like they were seriously ill. They did not look fit while losing weight.

They looked weak and frail because most of their weight loss was water and, worse, muscle mass.

Let's compare it to my friends and I who lost some weight but didn't look fit at all. How is this possible when I haven't lost as much "weight" as my diet-only friends? This was because while I was losing a lot of body fat, I was also building muscle mass at the same time. That's why I look fitter and stronger, even though I've lost less weight.

And when it comes to resistance or strength training, please don't think that you have to be a power lifter or bodybuilder or do your strenuous workout. These guys and gals are extreme, and chances are your body can't handle it. All you need to do is perform basic compound lifts like deadlifts, bench presses, and squats with enough weight.

Do 3 sets of 8 repetitions for each weightlifting exercise for optimal muscle training. My recommendation at this point is to train according to HFT (high frequency training). If you don't have access to a gym or set of weights, you can do bodyweight exercises like plyometrics and calisthenics instead. Your body is a good weight to work with. Start with the number of reps you can do for each exercise and gradually build up to 12 reps per set, requiring a minimum of 2 sets per exercise.

Chapter 11: Top Mistakes to Avoid

Getting things right is only half the battle. The other half is avoiding the mistakes that can ruin your success, especially the critical ones. And when it comes to intermittent fasting for weight loss, health, and energy, it's the same. Therefore, in this final chapter, we're going to discuss the top mistakes that can keep you from succeeding in temporary fasting and how to avoid them.

Eat the wrong foods

Many people who claim to have faithfully followed the guidelines and protocols of intermittent fasting do not have the appropriate results. Why is that, considering they reportedly kept their fasting and eating windows? If you asked them what they typically eat during their mealtime, you would be shocked to hear their answers: They mainly eat processed and unhealthy foods. There is a saying: garbage in, garbage out. When it comes to getting in great shape and health, nothing else is so true.

What you eat will ultimately determine how you look and feel. No intermittent fasting protocol is ever going to work for you if you just eat crap. Yes, there are some very talented people who seem exempt from this trash-eat-trash body curse. And those are the few exceptions to the rule. So please don't assume for a second that you are one of them. Unless there is compelling evidence that you are. You should be very careful about the foods you eat regularly and you shouldn't leave your diet to chance.

So what does it look like to eat healthy? On the one hand, healthy eating means that mainly whole or "natural" foods are eaten. Food that is as close to its original state as possible. The further a food is processed, the further it is from its original form, the more unhealthy ingredients have been added, many of which not only hold fat but also make you sick in the long run. What do whole foods look like? Grilled chicken, steak, and pork chops are natural or whole foods because they haven't changed from their original shape. On the flip side, burgers, hot dogs, and chicken nuggets are some of the best examples of processed foods that you need to minimize consumption for health and fitness purposes. Other examples of highly processed foods include bagels, donuts, cookies ... and the list goes on! Another type of food that you need to minimize or even avoid entirely are foods and drinks filled with sugar. Not only are they high calorie-dense - lots of calories for little volume - you put yourself at risk of slow metabolism and diabetes. Stick to plain water, green tea or unsweetened coffee for drinks and fruits, vegetables and brown rice for carbohydrates instead.

So much free time

There is a saying that idle hands are the devil's workshop. In a practical sense, it's true because when you have that much time on your hands you will tend to fill them with whatever is within reach. Because people are not there to do nothing - we will always look for something to fill our time. And often the closest, or most convenient, way to fill free time is through sedentary activities and eating. Worse, scrap and processed foods are the most convenient types. One of the best ways to minimize your risks to falling into this trap is to start your intermittent fast on a day that you think will be very active.

If you do, your mind will become too preoccupied with all of the things you need to do to the point that it is no longer aware of the major dietary changes. If you start your intermittent fasting journey at home on a lazy day, the risk of breaking the fast prematurely on the first day is high because most, if not all, of your attention is focused on nothing but your hunger.

Overdose of stimulants

Caffeine has been scientifically proven to help optimize physical and mental performance by, among other things, increasing your heart rate and making you feel awake. As a result, intermittent fasting can also help you burn more body fat. But while it can be a great thing, any good or great thing can be harmful once ingested in excess. A cup or two of unsweetened black coffee or green tea can be very helpful during the day, but drinking 3 or more regularly isn't very helpful.

Due to its acidic nature, drinking excessive caffeine can make you feel a lot hungrier than you really are, and can make it really difficult for you to stick to your fast.
Too much caffeine will also rob you of your night's sleep, which is even more important if you are fasting intermittently.

Lack of good sleep will make you feel weak, sluggish, and cloudy during the day, all of which greatly increase your risk of overcompensation - you guessed it right - eat! As a good general guideline, your last cup should be no later than 3pm. This should give your body enough time to flush the caffeine out of your system so that you can get a good night's sleep.

Set goals that are too high

Another way that you can fail before you start intermittent fasting is to set unrealistic goals for your fast. If you do that, you will fail. When it comes to achieving personal goals, set smaller, more realistic goals that focus on your most important ones. But these goals must also be challenging. Why? If they are not challenging, it means nothing to you, and that means you are not being encouraged to pursue the next higher goals. When you set smaller, realistic, and challenging goals, you can see small but big victories that build your confidence to achieve bigger goals.

What about intermittent fasting? Instead of trying to fast straight for 16 hours, your first goal should be to skip one main meal each day, lunch or dinner. If that's too big for you, try to skip snacks first before heading to main meals.

That way you won't shock your body. And as you gradually increase the length of your fasts, you build your capacity and confidence to fast for much longer periods of time.

Another example is weight loss. If you need to lose 25 pounds total, don't make it your goal to lose 25 pounds right away. Start with your goal of losing 5 pounds over 2 months first. Once you've done that, aim for the next 5 pounds, and so on, until you finally reach 25 pounds.

Afraid of an empty stomach

The greatest fear of many dieters, especially those adopting the intermittent fasting lifestyle, is the fear of being hungry as if it were the devil's child. Hunger is just another part of normal daily life and contrary to what many nutrition and fitness gurus preach, intermittent fasting does not lead to muscle wasting or loss when done correctly.

You will also not die prematurely after 24 hours of fasting unless you have fasted for 30 days! As mentioned in Chapter 1, it can make sense to use the right intermittent fasting protocols to get hungry in a targeted manner, which can have a very positive effect on your health and general fitness. If intermittent fasting is a surefire way to shrink your muscles and starve to death, why does regular or intermittent fasting play a huge role in the lives of millions of people around the world who are still alive, awake, alert, and enthusiastic are?

Continuously hungry after excessive periods of time is unhealthy or even downright dangerous. But that's not intermittent fasting. The word "intermittent" means, among other things, sporadic, irregular or erratic. In other words, intermittent implies something that is not continuous or long lasting. It's a stop-and-go thing. If you starve intermittently, you will not go to extreme starvation.

Be overly careful

There is an important principle in funding - especially investment - that can also be applied to intermittent fasting. If you want to get higher returns or profits, you need to take higher risks or more volatility. And according to Mr. Hofmekler (remember the glory of the Warrior Diet?), Volatility is your best friend when it comes to effective intermittent fasting.

To cut all the technical hocus-pocus, Hofmekler claims that the nutrients you ingest or ingest become even more beneficial or powerful if your body doesn't get them on a regular basis. When you start intermittent fasting, you are actually breaking the predictable nutrient consumption pattern that your body has been used to practically all of your life. And with this unpredictability, bigger results come. Looking at "hunger" in a negative light can be overly careful and avoid it at all costs.

But as with many investments, if you want to get bigger returns, you need to take bolder and riskier steps. In this case, you need to put down some of your personal walls that can keep you from sporadically targeted hunger.

If you take the risk of getting hungry on purpose, you are breaking your body's predictable eating pattern, thereby significantly increasing the nutritional benefits it gets from the foods you eat.

Much ado about timelines

No doubt about it - the length of your fast and how you schedule it are important aspects of intermittent fasting. But that doesn't mean you should be obsessed with timing because when you do it can only stress you out and negate or reduce your chances of achieving your fitness and health goals through intermittent fasting.

You should take it seriously, no doubt about it, but you shouldn't overdo it. You also need to learn to relax. So how can you tell if you're obsessed with timelines? If you are easily stressed out about instances where you are unable to fast or eat at your "right" times, then you probably are. While you should do your best to stick to your set fasting and fasting times, minutes after minutes will not derail your efforts to lose body fat and achieve great health.

Viewing individual components instead of the overall picture

The word synergy implies that the whole is greater than the sum of its parts. What does this mean for the layman? With synergy, 5 plus 5 equals 15!

Without synergy or using the simple arithmetic method, 5 plus 5 is just 10, which is the sum of its parts. When it comes to intermittent fasting, the beneficial results are due to the synergistic interactions of the various aspects. Intermittent fasting doesn't work per aspect or component - they work as a team. It's a holistic endeavor. Focus on just one or two components, e.g. B. Fasting, feeding, or hydrating, you won't get very far. You can only be very disappointed if you fail to achieve your weight loss and health goals and, as a result, bury the whole thing. So when you fast intermittently, always remember that it is about the synergy between the key components of fasting, meal times, meal time, quality of food, hydration, adequate sleep, regular exercise, and the inclusion of important practices.

When you look at the bigger picture, you will become less obsessed with each component and increase your chances of sticking to your chosen protocol and achieving your weight loss and health goals.

A "diet" perspective

Intermittent fasting is not just a "diet", it is a lifestyle. What that means is that it isn't something that you just try for a few weeks or months before going back to your previous eating habits. It's a way of life. When you look at it from such a short-term perspective, you are making two more mistakes that can sabotage your efforts to achieve your desired body weight and health.

The first of these mistakes is that when you are better at intermittent fasting you can go to extremes and neglect other important areas of your life such as family, friends, and work, among others. This can cause you to miss out on many of life's greatest joys and if you do you will eventually blame intermittent fasting for it and give it up completely. The second mistake you can make is by viewing intermittent fasting as a diet, rather than a healthy eating lifestyle, and causing you to have binge eating as soon as you are done with the diet.

And in most cases, people who eat right after a successful diet tend to not only regain the weight they lost, but also gain their previous weight. When you engage in intermittent fasting as a lifestyle, you will inadvertently consider all of the other important aspects of a healthy lifestyle and increase your chances of not only fasting for the long term, but also achieving your fitness and health goals. Take small steps and gradually relate to the intermittent fasting lifestyle. Doing this will increase your chances of successfully incorporating it into your lifestyle and keeping it there. And of course, you increase your chances of getting the most important benefits - healthy weight loss and good health.

Conclusion

As you have learned in this book, intermittent fasting is one of the best ways to get in good shape and health. You also learned the different types of intermittent fasting - protocols among others - and found that regardless of your personal circumstances or schedule, you can incorporate them as part of your overall lifestyle. The only exception would be if you have a pre-existing medical condition or special dietary needs. In addition, intermittent fasting can be a sustainable eating lifestyle that can greatly contribute to a fulfilling life.

But knowledge is only half the battle to losing weight and achieving good health. The other half is action or application of knowledge. Therefore, I strongly encourage you to apply what you have learned in this book as soon as possible. And as I've mentioned in a few chapters, you don't have to do everything at once.

Take small steps and gradually relate to the intermittent fasting lifestyle. Doing this will increase your chances of successfully incorporating it into your lifestyle and keeping it there. And of course, you increase your chances of getting the most important benefits - healthy weight loss and good health. Here is your success, my friend! Bottom up!

Please leave a review on Amazon if you found this book helpful.!

Book # 2: Burning Fat on Your Belly

Have you ever wondered why you aren't losing weight even though you are doing the exercises advised by self-appointed experts? **The truth is,** you can do as many exercises as you want, if you don't follow the 3-factor rule, you won't get results. Worse still, the effort will make you eat even more and gain weight! My name is John Dexter and I have been involved in professional fitness and strength training sports since I was 16. As a nutritionist and personal trainer, I can tell you that most of the books out there give false information. *Every book that tells you that you can specifically burn fat on your stomach lies to you!*

That's a fact! Our body decreases differently all over the body, it starts from top to bottom. I don't want to go into too much detail here and will get straight to the point.

If you do not exercise with a certain diet, or rather, diet, you will not lose weight! What does this mean for you and what do you have to do in order to lose weight successfully?

Well, we'll clear that all up in my 3-IN-1 book. I will give you the exercises, the diet and the recipes you need to do to be successful! You get the best of 3 worlds and can see results after just 7 days. It is the ultimate weight loss book.

Who is this book for?

Are you struggling with this dreaded "middle age range" or with an unsightly "muffin top"?
Do you also carry extra weight that always builds up around your stomach and hips? Are you struggling to find clothes that fit because your tummy is preventing you from fastening the buckle or zipper, and your mids are getting bigger and rounder? Would you also like to have a slim, beautiful stomach where you can easily see the abdominal muscles? Do you want a slim waist and a dream body?

If so, this book is for you!

Stop wasting time dieting that doesn't target your stubborn belly fat and boring sit-ups that only hurt your back or build strong muscles around your abdominal area.

If you're ready to lose belly fat, tone your tummy, and finally have the flattering figure you've always wanted, *then this book is for you!*

What will this book teach you? There's a reason people use the word "persistent" a lot when they talk about losing belly fat, because the fat around the middle is often the hardest to lose no matter what diet or exercise you try.

You've probably noticed that your middle keeps growing over time, and especially when you've reached middle age. The good news is that if you follow a few simple tips over dinner and while exercising, you can shed those stubborn pounds and inches around your midriff and create a slim and toned look.

You can target your abs with simple but effective exercises, and lose your fat with the right foods so that you get a well-shaped figure that will delight you. You can lose unwanted pounds while building firm muscle and toning your stomach, waist, and even your back. In this book we will tell you everything that you need to change in your diet, which exercises you need to do that are more effective than boring sit-ups and crunches to specifically lose your belly fat. Because remembering all of the tips and pointers you need to follow to burn that stubborn belly fat and tone the sculpted muscles around your waist can be a little overwhelming, we're going to break it down into 31 easy steps. So, when you're ready to work on your lean and toned abs to finally get the strong, lean abs you want, let's get started! 9

Why belly fat is so stubborn and so difficult to lose

Before we talk about how we lose that belly fat, let's first talk about why your body is clinging to this fat in the first place, and why it is so hard to lose. This can help you understand why some of these techniques will be successful, and why certain diets or exercise exercises that you have tried in the past may have let you down over the years.

Why do you get fat?

First, notice how and why the body gets excess fat in the first place. Your body weight is a ratio between the calories you consume and the calories you burn from physical activity. This activity includes the day-to-day functioning of your systems like heartbeat, lung breathing and so on. When you take in more calories than you use, those calories are converted and then stored as fat by your body. These fat stores are tapped and converted back into energy if you don't eat enough calories to support your activities.

This may suggest that it is easy to burn off those fat reserves with just a little exercise or following a new diet. But keep in mind that the body uses the glucose from the foods you eat before it uses up those fats.

The body also needs to burn a ton of calories before you can see any significant difference.

That doesn't mean you should starve to lose weight, but it does explain why losing weight is so hard. You can't just cut a few calories here and there and expect to lose enough weight.

Why is the belly fat?

Losing weight on the stomach is also the most difficult because it forces the body to hold onto most of the stored fat. The abdomen is a safe place to store those extra pounds without putting unnecessary strain on your muscles. If the body was storing excess fat around your legs or arms, you would soon feel muscle fatigue every time you used your arms and legs. Storing a lot of fat on your back can also increase your risk of injuring your back muscles every time you stand up or lie on your back.

The body burns most of the fat from the other places before it turns to the fat stores on the abdomen to reduce the stress it is putting on the muscles by storing the added fat. You can see your arms, back, breasts, and even your face get slimmer as you lose weight while your tummy is still a problem for your favorite jeans!

Because most of your stored fat is trapped around your stomach, you won't even notice if you've lost weight on your stomach. You can easily see the difference on your arms, legs, back, and other such places as you start burning pounds, but you may not notice it around your stomach anytime soon. You can, however, measure your stomach or check your clothes to see whether you have lost weight on your stomach. It's also good to weigh yourself regularly as you lose weight and gain muscle, but keep in mind that a body fat indicator can be an even better tool for tracking your progress. You could actually lose belly fat while building muscle, so the scales could be a poor indicator of your progress too.

Exercise the stomach

Exercising the abs can also be difficult as the body will likely use the back muscles and leg muscles when exercising before activating the abs. With the right exercises, you can train your abs that are more effective than the everyday sit-ups as many people get them wrong by using the back and leg muscles. Simple exercises that use the body's own weight for resistance and specifically target the abdominal muscles can tighten and shape the abdominal muscles with just a few repetitions and little strain.

Now that you know a little more about how the body creates and stores fat, and why losing it around your belly is such a challenge, let's start looking at the best ways to melt that fat away. We're going to first discuss some changes to your diet that can help you cut calories, and then we'll discuss some of the foods you can take to aid your muscle building routine.

These foods will also help you cut empty calories from your diet and ensure that you are healthier overall. Then we're going to do a few simple exercises and everyday activities that you can do to tone and tone the core. We're going to go through them carefully so that you can do them properly. In no time you will have firm and toned abs and a lean and muscular figure.

Tip 1: Count calories

One very important thing that you can do to burn belly fat is to keep track of your calories. Since body fat is converted from calories that you have ingested but not burned, reducing your caloric intake can turn your body into its own fat burning machine. When you cut down on your calories, your body will be forced to turn to these fat stores for energy. However, you cannot realize the need to cut your calories unless you want to keep track of how much you are consuming and you do not want to dangerously cut your calories so that you will starve.

Keeping track of what you are eating, how much, how many calories it contains, and all these other details is a very good step in reducing those calories while staying healthy and safe. Counting calories isn't as hard as you might think. You can even use a simple app on your smartphone to add up your calories throughout the day and then transfer those numbers to a calendar or spreadsheet.

If you don't have a smartphone, use a simple little notebook that you keep in a pocket or purse and write down what you eat throughout the day. Each night add these calories on your calendar and you'll see where some cuts can be made.

One very important note: you need to be honest with yourself when tracking what you eat and drink. Often we are not honest with ourselves and estimate the calorie consumption during the day less than it actually is:

- If you compare a heaped tablespoon of sugar versus a level tablespoon, that's probably the same as two tablespoons of sugar.
- Don't overlook small things like cream in your coffee, vinegar on your salad, or a piece of butter that you put on your vegetables. The same goes for small pieces of candy, a few peanuts, raisins, or other foods that aren't high in calories per serving. Add these to your calorie count, even if you suspect it is no more than 10 or 20 calories that you are consuming with each bite.

- Canned and packaged foods have a nutritional table. But these are per serving, and it can contain two or even more servings per packet. One serving of soup that you take has 200 calories. However, the can can have a total of 400 or more calories; Make sure you read the labels and write down the serving size, not just the calorie count.

- The only zero calorie foods are water, coffee, and diet soda! Don't think that you need other "diet" foods that are low in sugar or low-fat foods that do not count towards your calories. Even fruits, vegetables, and other such foods should be included as these calories can add up over time.

- Stay honest about foods that aren't exactly portioned for you and stay on the caution side. As an example of what this means when you have a fast food lunch with a friend, check the calorie count of certain foods on the restaurant's website or elsewhere.

If you eat your own burger and then eat the final bites of your friend's burger, be sure to write down the calories from your own burger, but should also add some extra calories to your record to include the bites of your friend's meal!

- Don't forget to add whatever you drink to your calorie intake, including juices, tea, flavored coffee, and milk.

Once you start counting calories, you need to compare the calories you are consuming to a healthy amount for your gender, age, and overall physical fitness. You may actually be surprised at how many calories you are realistically consuming each day and realizing that some changes need to be made to reduce belly fat.

If you're not sure how to cut the calories on your own, next let's discuss some small steps you can take to cut those calories and get your body to turn to those fat stores for energy.

Tip 2: brush off the sugar

Sugar has no nutritional value at all. It doesn't contain proteins, vitamins, trace elements, amino acids, or anything your body needs for general health. In truth, sugar only has "empty calories" and is only used to sweeten foods. This is why not consuming pure sugar is one of the best ways to see the fat go away around your stomach area. Once you stop consuming sugar or reduce it drastically, you will be consuming far fewer calories and you may eventually lose those unwanted pounds. These simple changes mean cutting down on calories without having to count them.

Pay attention to where most of the sugar is in your diet so you know where to start e.g. B:

- Sugar in your coffee

- Sugar in the muesli
- Sugary sodas and sweetened teas.
- Energy drinks
- frozen desserts such as ice cream and milkshakes or iced coffee
- Fruit juices with added sugar
- cookie
- cake
- Candy bars and other sweets
- Canned fruits in fruit syrup
- bottled salad dressings
- granola bar
- Breakfast bars
- Protein bars and shakes

To reduce your belly fat, make a note of how many of them you have in your daily diet and remove them from your diet entirely. Consider some ways to make changes to your diet so that you still have the foods you love, but without all of those extra sugars:

- Try flavored coffee beans instead of flavored creamer.
- Make your own fruit juice at home by mixing filtered water and fresh fruit.
- Unsweetened iced tea with fresh lemon instead of sweetened tea.
- Add fresh fruit to a low-sugar muesli or a low-sugar yogurt variant to your breakfast.
- Opt for fresh fruit instead of canned fruit.

- Make your own salad dressing by whipping skimmed milk with flavor packs or switch to the vinegar and oil dressing.
- Make trail mix with peanuts, desiccated coconut, and a few raisins to replace the place of your granola bars.

These substitutes are all much lower in their sugar content and still give you the nutrients you need and a touch of sweetness you want in your foods. At this point I would like to recommend a book by James Wilson "Living Sugar Free and Ending Sugar Addiction"

Tip 3: Cut down on simple carbohydrates

There are many misconceptions about carbohydrates and how they affect your body weight, as well as when and why you need to remove them to lose belly fat in particular. The right carbohydrates in your diet can actually help you lose belly fat, while lowering other carbohydrates can help burn that stubborn fat. To understand how and why carbohydrates can help reduce your belly fat, let's take a closer look at carbohydrates as a whole.

Simple and complex carbohydrates

Carbohydrates are considered simple or complex. Complex carbohydrates are made from whole grains and have minimal, if any, processing. Simple carbohydrates were processed to remove some or most of that grain. These grains that are processed are often called white flour, so the most common simple carbohydrates source in your foods made from white flour. This includes all types of pasta, bread, cookies and muffins, cakes, biscuits, crackers, pretzels and other similar baked goods and snacks, pancakes and waffles, pizza dough and other such foods.

Why are you reducing or removing simple carbohydrates?

The reason simple carbohydrates should be removed from your diet is because they are processed into a form of sugar in the body. When this sugar isn't absorbed into the body's bloodstream and then used for energy, it becomes part of all of the body's stored fat. So eating lots of simple carbohydrates will not help you lose fat. On the contrary, it adds some!

Simple carbohydrates are also typically very high in calories, which means you are getting very little nutrition for the amount of calories you are eating. Think how many calories are in crackers and pretzels, as well as bread and pasta, and watch how they are easily added to that belly fat, even though they are not necessarily made with a lot of added sugar.

When removing foods that add to your belly fat, start with pasta, white bread, and baked goods. This includes crackers, pretzels, and other such snacks. Eliminate these from your diet completely and you can see some pounds and inches begin to melt away.

Anything made with a white flour batter should typically be removed, including pizza, hamburger and hot dog buns and noodles in the soup. These are all simple carbohydrates and will not help you burn belly fat!

Tip 4: Avoid starchy foods

Starchy foods include potatoes, lima beans, rice, corn, and peas. The starch in these foods is a form of carbohydrate, so it is also broken down as sugar in the body. These types of sugar don't give you a lot of energy, will help put on even more pounds if you're not active enough to burn that sugar before it can be turned into fat. These foods, like other foods high in carbohydrates, are also very high in calories so you won't get a lot of nourishment for the amount of calories you consume. This is why you should avoid starchy foods to melt away the stubborn belly fat.

The challenge is that many people have starchy foods as the main staple in their diet, potatoes are often served as fries for lunch and then as a side dish at dinner.

Fried potatoes can also be part of a hot breakfast. Corn is often served as a side dish, mixed with beans or ground to many meals to make tortillas and other bread substitutes. Rice is also a staple food for many people and their daily diet. Adding honey, sugar, and other such high-calorie sweeteners to rice also make it a very unhealthy dish when it comes to melting body fat. By making a list of the starchy foods you have during the week, you can see where some cuts can be made.

Don't assume that potatoes are an important part of dinner and switch to oats instead of rice. At dinner, try other vegetable side dishes like broccoli, cauliflower, asparagus, or green beans. These foods have little to no starch and will help you fill yourself up so you can better control your appetite and melt away that stubborn belly fat.

Tip 5: Reduce fruit

Fruit is very healthy because it contains many vitamins, trace elements, and other nutrients that you need to be healthy. The hydration of fruits can also leave you feeling full and satisfying your sweet tooth when you skip on pure sugars. Fruit is also easy to take with you when you need to bring a snack to the office or elsewhere, and is a great substitute for candy bars and other sugary treats. Then why cut down on fruit when you want to lose belly fat?

The reason is that fruits have a high concentration of sugars that can add to your daily calorie count and add those pounds around your belly. While fruit can be healthier than baked goods, sweets, and other foods that are devoid of all of these nutrients, you can still get too much sugar if you eat a lot of fruit every day. The key to fruit is how much fruit you have each day in a healthy amount and make sure you have more vegetables instead of fresh fruit.

You also want a variety of fruits that aren't the highest concentration of sugar but still have all of these healthy nutrients. Fruits with the highest sugar content are apples and bananas. But fruits with the lowest amount of sugar are grapes, melons and berries of all varieties. To satisfy that sweet tooth and get the nutrients it needs from fruits, cut down on your bananas and apples and eat more mixed berries, watermelons, melons and grapes. They are great desserts with no added sweeteners or sugar.

You can add some berries to a protein shake and get a taste of sweetness along with your needed nutrients without having too much sugar from fruits every day. Also, keep in mind that sugar from fruits is also found in fruit juice. Even if no sugar has been added to the juice, you can get quite a number of calories and sugars from fruit juice alone.

Make your own juice by mixing filtered water and healthy berries so you can control how much fruit is mixed in and make sure no sugar is added. Add a little lemon or lime with a little sugar, but very tasty, for an extra flavor.

Tip 6: Eat more fiber

A calorie deficit will help you burn fat on your stomach, but you should also consider food choices. One of those particular foods is fiber. Fiber Will Really Help You Lose Weight! There are a couple of reasons why fiber is so important for weight loss. One of them is that they spread in your stomach and fill you up. In return, you will eat less. This will make it easier for you to control your calories.

Fiber takes a long time to digest, so you may experience less hunger and cravings between meals, and you can also control your daily calorie intake. Fiber also binds to other foods and helps break them down, making it much easier for them to move through the digestive system. Also, the chances of getting gas from foods with fiber will decrease, and your bowel movements will be easier. Also, when food is able to move better through your digestive system, it can mean the body is not absorbing glucose and sugar and converting them to fat.

Fiber is also not as high in calories as other foods, so you can eat more of it without consuming any calories. A bowl of oatmeal usually has a lot fewer calories than a bowl of sugary cereal!

Where is fiber found?

A fiber is an herbal product and is only found in plant-based foods including vegetables and oats. Whole grains are very high in fiber, as are leafy green vegetables. Look for a variety of lettuce, broccoli, cauliflower, beans, and asparagus if you want to add fiber to your diet. Add more oatmeal to breakfast, whole grain breads, and lots of salads. The peel of fruit is usually high in fiber too, so don't peel apples, eat oranges with their pulp instead of drinking orange juice with the pulp removed. All of these high fiber foods can help you control your eating and cut down on the calories you need to finally lose belly fat.

Tip 7: Drink plenty of water

Water can be one of the best things to put into your system for losing belly fat. There are many benefits to drinking water when it comes to your overall health. One benefit is that water saturates you so you can eat less. Having a glass of water before meals can mean you can eat less and feel full. In fact, when you think you are hungry, you may just be dehydrated and the body is trying to get some fluids and hydration, which is provided by food, not just water.

Water also helps optimize the digestive system with other foods so you have fewer problems with elimination and you don't feel bloated. Water also nourishes your blood and makes it easier for the body to circulate the blood. This is necessary in order to provide muscles with the important proteins and amino acids they need to become strong. If you are exercising to get a tight and lean stomach, you need water to build healthy muscles!

Drinking water also helps the body reduce belly fat, making it easier for the fat cells to break open when the body needs energy. It also flushes out toxins when you urinate, making you feel less sluggish and tired and have more energy.

How to Drink More Water Every Day

To be able to drink more water, consider these practical tips:

- Schedule a time to drink a glass or half a glass of water each day. This could be every hour on the hour. You can also make it part of your daily routine, have a glass of water after you get to the office or right after lunch, right after you get home and right after your favorite evening program. If you create a schedule for yourself, the more likely you will continue to drink water.
- Always have a bottle of water with you even if you think you are not going to drink it. If you always have a bottle with you, you'll drink it too, and every sip helps!

- Throw in some lemon or lime slices or a few cherries or other berries if the water is a bit boring for you.

A little flavor can make water more palatable, and a few small pieces of fresh fruit shouldn't add too much to your daily calorie content.
- Have your water in two 1 liter bottles and do not end your day until you have drunk the water in both bottles. Keep one bottle in the refrigerator to keep it cool and swap it out when the other bottle warms up. You can also use a water jug for fresh filtered water. Fill it up at night and keep it in the fridge, don't go to bed the next day until all the water is gone.

Tip 8: Eat more protein

Protein is important in building a lean and toned stomach because protein is a building block of muscle. If you are not getting enough protein in your diet, you can do any exercise you want and still not have strong muscles. Many people assume that you can only get protein from meat and dairy products, but this is not true. There is a lot of protein in certain vegetables and foods like soy. While protein is important, don't forget the extra calories you can get from saturated fat in many animal products such as beef, cheese, and butter. These foods are high in protein, but also high in calories.

Instead, opt for lean sources of protein:

- Chicken, Turkey and Fish
- Beans and especially black beans
- Peanuts and peanut butter
- Soy products
- Dark leafy vegetables
- Eggs
- legumes

Consider the many options and incorporate these foods into your diet. Legumes like chickpeas can be ground and mixed with garlic, lemon, and olive oil to make homemade hummus. Soy can contain soy milk and tofu, which are often found in meatless casseroles. You can also choose a type of nut milk such as cashew or almond milk instead of milk. Add spinach to an omelette and you have both eggs and dark leafy greens on one plate!

Tip 9: Stretching

Let's move on to the exercises you can do to shape and strengthen your stomach. Stretching is a very simple exercise and movement, but very beneficial for the abdomen. The more you stretch, the more blood and healing oxygen your muscles will receive so they can get stronger and leaner. You can do whatever you want to your stomach without stretching, your muscles will never be lean, tight and not look nice and tight. Stretching can also help improve your posture, as you are more likely to stand erect and straight when your muscles are properly stretched.

When muscles, bones, and joints are not stretched, they tend to bend over themselves and become tense, but stretching actually elongates muscles and tendons. In return, you will look slimmer because you won't be slumped.

Stretching in practice especially for the stomach

To stretch your abs, you need to use movements that specifically target the middle. A good yoga pose that you could try is called the cobra position:

1. Lie on your stomach with your hands next to your shoulders, palms flat on the floor as if you were doing a push-up.

2. However, instead of lifting your torso straight up in the air, arch up and backward. Start by lifting your face, then your neck, then your shoulders, then your torso off your exercise mat and use your hands for balance. Make sure the back is curved in an inverted C shape.

3. You will feel your back muscles curve inward as your abs curve upward and outward. Lower yourself back down on the mat by stretching backwards

again. Lower your stomach, then torso, then shoulders then neck, then head.

4. After a short rest, repeat this position and hold this curve as long as possible.

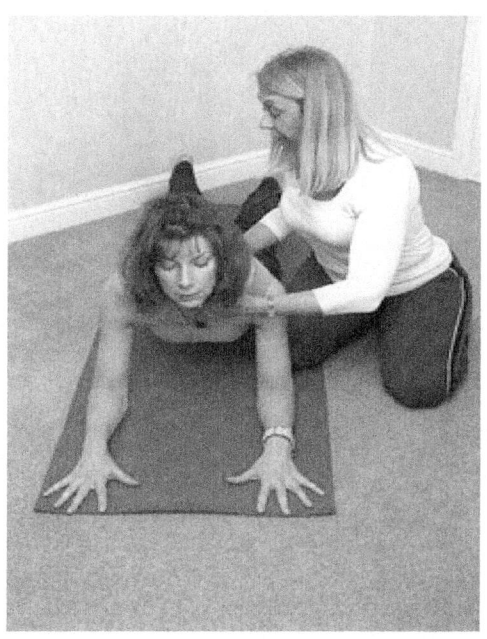

Another easy step is to stand with your feet shoulder-width apart.

1. Keeping your balance and making sure that your weight is evenly supported, then close your hands over your head or place them on the back of your hips.

2. Gently straighten your entire back in a C shape and keep your arms on your hips or reach behind you for a deeper stretch.

3. Feel the abdominal muscles stretch. Gently to the left and then to the right for an even deeper

stretch. Instead of swinging in this position, slowly and simply stretch yourself.

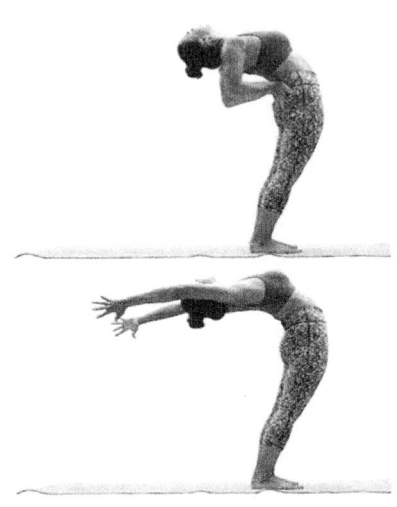

Tip 10: Simple leg lifts

To work out the abs and make sure you are targeting them, try a simple leg lift.

1. Lie on the exercise mat, on your back, with your legs together and stretched out, arms by your sides.

2. Raise your legs just a few inches off the floor, keeping your feet together. Don't put your hands on the floor for leverage as you want the abs to do the work of keeping your legs up in the air. Also, don't lift your legs more than a few inches, because if you hold them at an angle of 45 degrees or higher, you

will be supported by the back and hip muscles and your abs won't work as hard. Just hold them up a few inches and you will feel your abs working!

3. You also don't want to pump your legs up and down as this puts stress on your back, and the momentum doesn't allow the abs to work properly either.

Just keep your feet a little off the floor and you will feel your abs work and tone up.

4. Put your feet back on the floor to rest them, then repeat this exercise keeping your feet up for as long as possible.

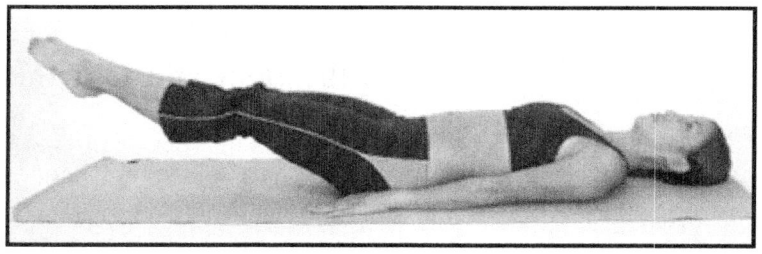

Tip 11: The 8 shape

Another step that specifically targets the abs is the 8 shape.

1. Lie on your back on the exercise mat and straighten your legs in the air so your body forms a 90-degree angle.

2. Keep your ankles together and your arms by your sides so you can't help, you want your abs to do the work.

3. Carefully make an 8th shape with your feet in the air toward the ceiling without keeping your feet wider than your hips or lower than your knees. Keep Figure 8 firm and compact. Do this four times in one direction and then four times in the opposite direction.

4. Lower your legs to the floor and rest, then come back and repeat this movement. Be sure to keep the number 8 small as it will do most of the work on your abs.

Your abs should be tight to control the movement of your legs during this exercise.

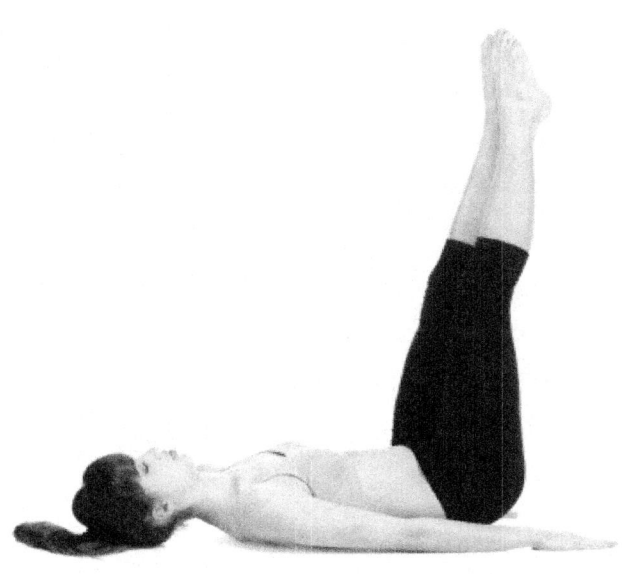

Tip 12: Roll like a ball

Rolling like a ball is a popular Pilates exercise and it affects the abdominal muscles and increases balance. It can also help loosen up some fat that you may be wearing on your back and tone your back.

>   1. Sit on your exercise mat and pull your legs up, knees to your chest.
>   2. Wrap your arms around your knees, then lift your feet straight off the floor. Your abs will tighten to

keep you balanced. This exercise itself is very good for working the abs. However, you can increase the challenge you give these muscles by rolling yourself slightly.

3. Lean to one side and then forward, to the other side, and back so that you form a circle with your body.

4. Make sure to keep your feet off the floor and keep the circle very small and tight so your abs have to work hard to make sure you can stay in this position.

If you roll too far forward, it can mean your back muscles are tightening, and if you roll too far back you can fall out of position.

5. Repeat this circle in one direction as many times as possible, then switch directions.

6. Put your feet on the floor and rest, then repeat. Make sure to keep your back straight and relaxed so that you are only using your abs and not your back to perform this movement.

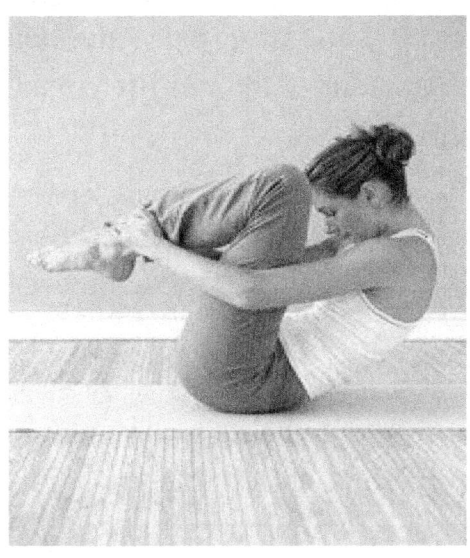

Tip 13: Semi sit-ups

One reason sit-ups and crunches are ineffective is because people often don't do them properly, and the movement causes them to lose tension so the stomach isn't working really hard. Your abs work the hardest when you lift your back and shoulders off the floor.

After that, the back and hip muscles begin to work so that you can finish your movement. To avoid this, try the half sit-ups.

1. To do this, lie on your back on the exercise mat. Put your feet under furniture if you have to, or bend your knees and keep your feet flat on the floor.

2. Put your hands behind your head or cross your arms under your neck and lift your upper body just a few inches.

3. You should now feel your abs tighten. Hold the position for a few seconds, then come back to the mat.

Repeat this movement but work slowly so that you are really focused and challenging the abs.

Do not lift your upper body more than a few inches off the floor and do not use your back muscles to hold yourself in position. You don't want to hunch over in this position either, but instead want to lift your body directly off the mat. Curling will keep the back muscles working, but if you keep your torso straight the abs will kick in to give you support. Because this movement keeps the abs tight and flexed, they target those muscles entirely, so you can get a better workout than crunches and sit-ups.

Tip 14: Reverse sit-ups

The abs can be worked when you are seated, but they also work hard to support your body when you recline from a seated position. To really challenge the muscles in this way, try reverse sit-ups.

1. To perform this exercise, sit on the mat and bend your knees with your feet flat on the floor.

2. Keep your hands clasped in front of you. Tighten your abs as you slowly return to the mat and feel these muscles struggle to keep you balanced and strong.

3. Do it like you're fighting your body as you lie on the mat, working your abs to keep you upright as you work to push yourself back off the mat.

4. Slowly go through this leaning back motion on the mat and your abs will work harder to keep your body from collapsing.

Try to keep still and not wobble, from this upright position, move slowly and fluidly back to the mat.

Remember to tense your abdominal muscles and keep your back relaxed so that the back muscles don't help at all! You also don't want to tense the leg muscles as they will also distribute some weight and effort, and you won't get the effective ab workout. If you did it right, you will feel the abs work extra hard to fight the movement and this will help you keep them toned and firm, better than a normal quick sit-up.

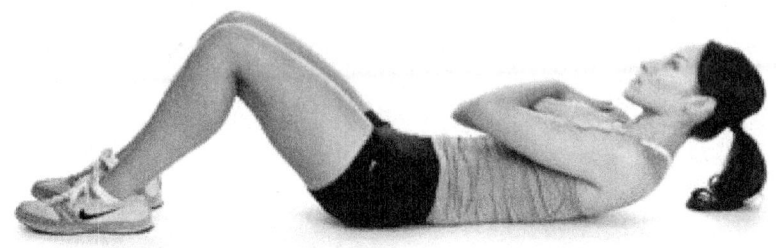

Tip 15: Reverse crunch

A variation on a reverse sit-up is the reverse crunch. This exercise is done without a chair or sofa to support your legs, but it is very challenging and can build abs faster than standard crunches.

1. To do the exercise, lie on your back on your mat with your hands behind your head or at your sides.
2. Raise your legs so they are straight in the air, your feet together, and your body is at a 90-degree angle.
3. Next, bend your knees slightly so that you can pull them toward you. Then use your abs to keep your torso on the mat, but pull your back end and hips off the floor so that your knees move even more toward you, your feet still up in the air. Don't pull

your legs too close to your body, just raise your back and hips so that your body curls up slightly.

4. Repeat this movement slowly and fluently with your abs to control your feet and legs, and lift your hips off the mat. Don't swing your legs back and forth as that swing takes away some of the work your abs have to do.

5. Focus on contracting your abs to bring your legs into position and then lie flat on the mat again. You also don't want to tense your shoulders and neck, as this can lead to muscle strain and pain. Isolate the abs for this movement and you will find them more effective than standard crunches.

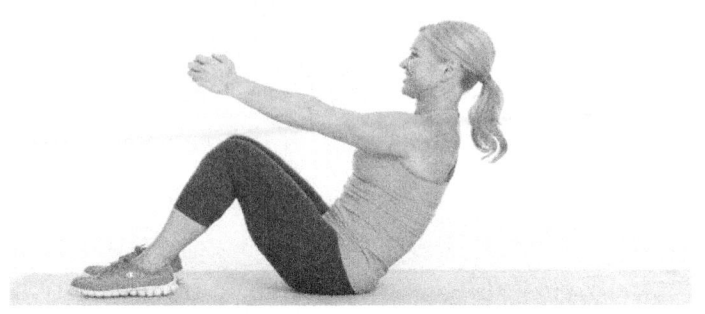

Tip 16: V-crunch

Another exercise that is similar to a crunch but is much more effective at targeting the abdomen is the V-crunch. This movement can tone and shape the abdomen, and even elongate and stretch the back muscles.

> 1. To do a V-crunch, lie on your back and then lift your legs in the air, straight up, so your body forms a 90-degree angle. Keep your feet together.
> 2. Your hands are not clasped behind your head during this exercise.
> 3. Keeping your hips and buttocks on the mat, lift your torso and straighten your arms in front of you as if trying to touch your toes. Don't pull your legs back.

This movement targets the abdominal muscles better than normal crunches. Keeping your legs in the air will make your abs work harder than if you were propping your feet under a piece of furniture.

Make sure you contract your abs so that you are working really hard and not lifting your back. Bring the body into the correct position and then bend back down, tensing the abdominal muscles all the time. Don't bob or move too fast, as slow and steady movement is the best way to challenge the abs.

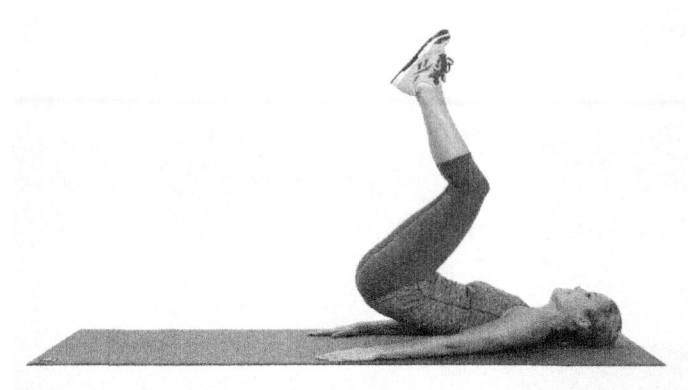

Tip 17: Plank

A plank can look very simple, but it really takes a lot of strain on the entire central area of the body. It can also help tone and tone the leg muscles and back.

1. Lie on your stomach.
2. Place your elbows and forearms on the mat and lift yourself up so that your elbows, forearms, and toes are the only parts of you on the mat.
3. Keep your body straight and stretched. Do not slump or curl your back while doing this. When you feel your back collapse or bend, slide your feet back or your arms forward a little so your body is in a long straight line.

4. Also, keeping your head in a straight line, look down at the floor as this will relieve the neck muscles.

5. Tighten your abs so they will work hard to keep you in this position.

6. Because the elbows and toes are the only parts of your body that hold your body weight, the abs will do everything they can to hold you. Hold this position for as long as possible before returning to the mat to rest. Then repeat the exercise.

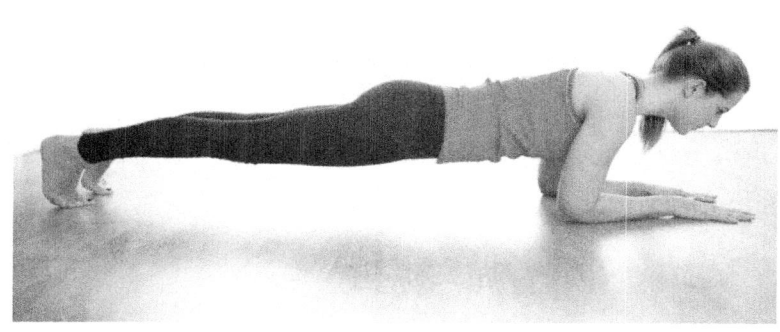

Tip 18: Crunch on the ball

An exercise ball gives you a number of ways to train your abs. The abs are worked more effectively when you use an exercise ball as your muscles work hard to keep you upright on the ball. The same exercise you did on the floor can be made in difficulty just by using an exercise ball!

> 1. Sit on the edge of the ball, feet flat on the floor, legs a little wider than shoulder width, fingers crossed behind your head.
> 2. Start by leaning back on the ball, then moving forward in a seated crunch. Make sure you contract your abs so that your back is not strained, and keep your feet on the floor so the ball does not roll out behind you or roll with you.
> 3. Keep your torso straight so your abs do the work. Do not rock back and forth, but do the exercise slowly and in a flowing movement so that the abdominal muscles are always tense.

You may need to try this exercise a few times to help you stay balanced and get used to it.

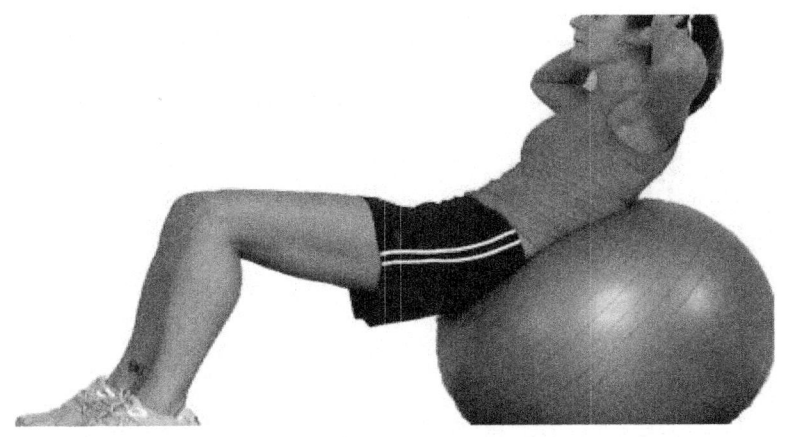

Tip 19: Roll the ball

This exercise is a little more difficult than the others, but it is good for aligning the abs and making them tone and firm.

1. To get into the right position, lie on the ball under the center of your stomach with your feet flat on the floor.

2. Roll your body forward onto the ball so you can reach the floor with your hands in front of you, your palms flat on the floor, and bring your legs onto the ball.

3. Either move forward with both hands or, if your abs are developed enough to move the exercise ball, move your legs backward. Do not raise your hands

as they need to stay on the floor while doing this movement.

4. Once in this position, keeping your hands flat on the floor, use your legs to roll the ball forward.

The abs will work to keep you balanced and secure as you move the ball back and forth with your ankles.

Be very careful as you can easily fall off the ball. However, once you learn how it works for you, you will feel your abs, legs, and back working hard.

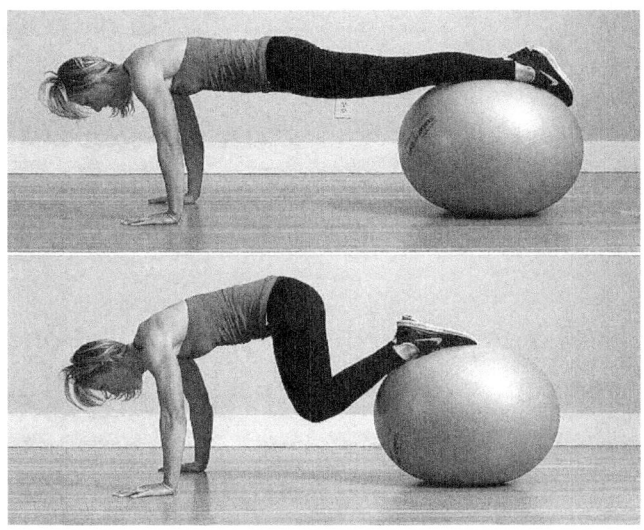

Tip 20: dumbbell front squat

Squats are designed to build up the back including the buttocks, thighs, and upper legs. When doing a squat, push up with the muscles in your legs and glutes. When you put a weight on your shoulders, either as free weights that you hold in your hands or as a dumbbell that you hold behind your neck and on your shoulders, it can be more of a challenge. While standard squats are intended to train the back, the front squats train the abdominal muscles as well as the glutes and legs.

1. Use a dumbbell, with or without weights, and hold it in front of your shoulders, balanced over the top of your chest, under your neck.
2. Now bend straight down until you reach a 90-degree angle.
3. Hold for a few seconds, then push yourself back up.
4. With dumbbells, make sure you keep your back straight, not leaning forward, and not lifting your back. You need to push up with your legs and back, using your heels instead of your toes.

When you do a squat, you contract your abs. Feel the stomach work to position the body. This will work out your entire midsection and back for a sleek, shapely look.

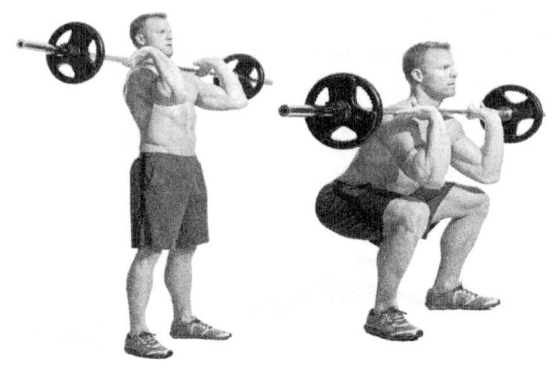

Tip 21: knee raises

Chine raises are like crunches, but they can be easier for those with back problems. In this exercise, you crunch with your lower body, not your upper body.

1. Lie on the floor with your legs in front of you, feet together.
2. Crunch forward so your back is at a 45-degree angle and place your hands behind your head to support yourself.
3. Pull your legs up off the mat while bending your knees outwards. Keep your feet together and touch

on the sides, but let your knees fall out slightly until they are only shoulder width apart.

Note that your feet should also be raised. You will feel your abs work to keep you balanced and upright.

You can hold your legs in this position for a few seconds, with your knees out and feet together to raise the level. Push your legs down, bring your knees back together, and repeat the exercise.

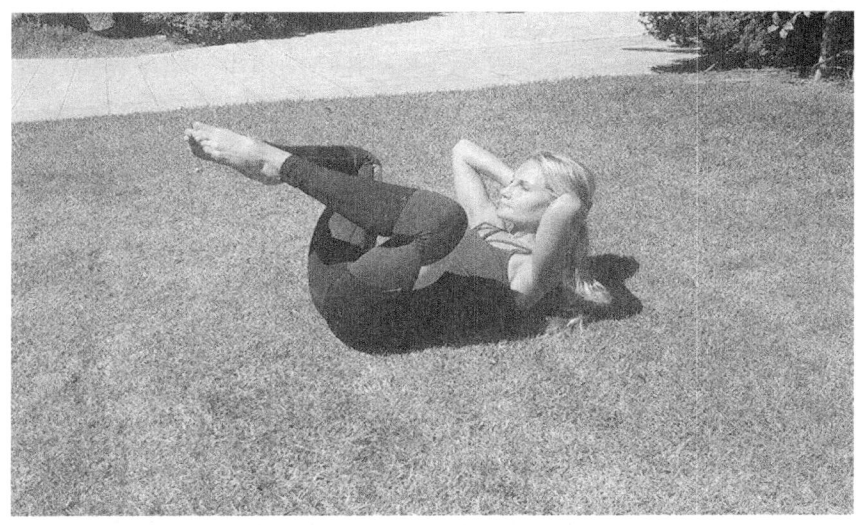

Tip 22: Hanging knee raises

A variation of the knee lift that is more challenging and that requires a bit more equipment is the hanging knee lift. You will need a pull-up bar for this exercise.

1. Hang on to the pole.
2. Now pull your legs up, either to your hips or your knees to your chest, and hold for a few seconds. Here you can also stretch your legs right in front of you. Both positions are very demanding and require the abdominal muscles to keep your body upright.

This exercise is more difficult than you might think and requires a little practice to be able to pull your legs up or in front of you. And you need enough arm strength to hang on to the bar. At the gym, you might find equipment that works more like a stand than a pull-up bar. This stand will have bars on either side that you can support your arms on.

You climb onto the stand, put your feet on a step and your arms on the bars, and then lift your legs up towards your chest or in front of you. If you find the hanging knee raise on the bar too difficult, try this equipment first until you have developed enough strength and coordination to hold onto the bar long enough.

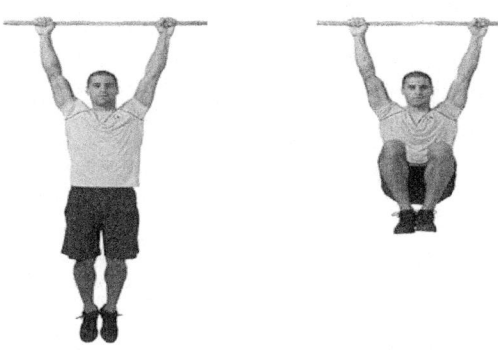

Tip 23: Side bends for the stomach

To get a nice belly, you should also work your side abs. This exercise ensures that you get a slim waist, the hourglass shape you want. This exercise looks simple and is certainly easy to do, but it is also a great challenge for your abs.

1. To do side bends, stand straight with your legs shoulder width apart.
2. Have a free weight in each hand. The amount of weight should be challenging but manageable.
3. Now slowly fiddle your body to the left as far as you can.
4. Keep the weight close to your body while doing this.

5. Now return to the starting position and repeat on the right side.

Go very slowly and do not bounce or bounce up and down, but let the muscles work slowly and effectively through the movement.

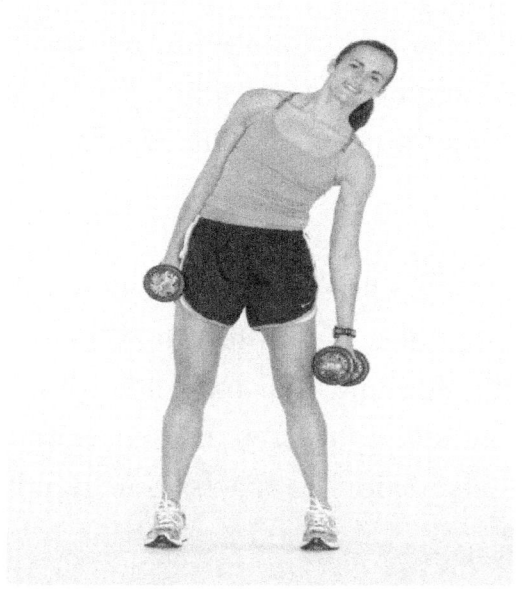

Tip 24: Russian twist

Another exercise that works the sides of the waist, but is a little more challenging, is called the "Russian Twist". For this exercise you will need a medicine ball, which is a weighted ball the size of a volleyball. Make sure it's a weighted ball. A basketball or volleyball won't work.

1. Sit on the floor, legs straight, feet together.
2. Holding the ball in your hands, then lift your feet off the floor, knees slightly bent.
3. Now turn around your hips, hold the ball in front of you, and then touch the floor on one side of you.

4. Now turn over on the other side and repeat the whole thing. Be sure to turn gently and not jump back and forth or pulsate with the movement as this will only irritate the muscles. Your abs will work hard to keep your legs balanced. The lateral muscles are also trained!

For a very challenging variation, do this movement with a friend, sitting back to back. If you turn to the side, your friend will also turn to the side and you hand them the ball. Repeat this turn for a count of eight or ten, then start on the other side. You need to twist deeper to reach your friend's hands, this makes the exercise very effective for the abs.

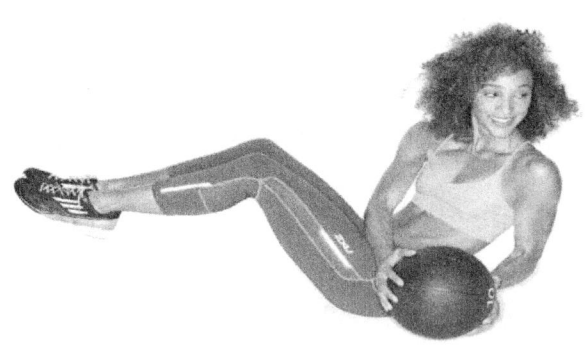

Tip 25: Bike crunch

The complete abdominal muscles are trained with the "bicycle crunch".

It also helps get blood circulation going and stretching your leg muscles for better posture and overall strength.

1. To perform this movement, lie down on the mat with your legs outstretched and your hands folded behind your head.

2. Raise your upper body halfway, no higher than a 45-degree angle, then also raise both legs so that your feet are only slightly off the floor.

3. Pull your left knee close to your chest and twist it so that your right elbow touches that knee.

4. Do the exercise in one smooth motion without lowering your back or legs on the mat, keeping your left leg straight, and bending your right knee by twisting in that direction so your left elbow touches your right knee.

You should move your legs in a slightly circular motion, like you would when riding a bicycle. Instead of rocking your torso back and forth, hold it in one place and twist it very gently while your opposite elbow touches each knee. Your abs will work hard to keep you in place and keep your legs moving.

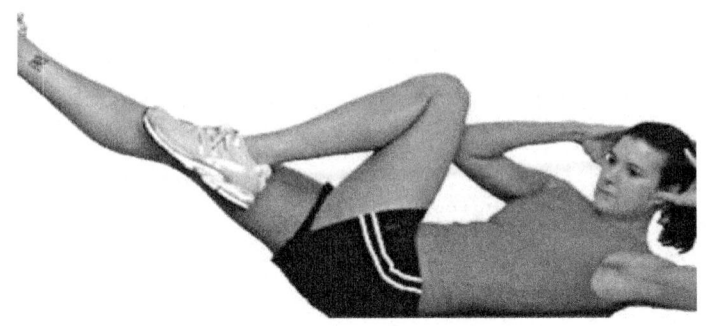

Tip 26: scissor lift

To get your legs off your exercise mat, your abs need to work hard. If you lie flat on your back, you can modify this simple movement for an even greater challenge. A scissor lift is very effective and easy.

1. Lift your legs off the floor just enough to feel your abs.
2. Next, spread your legs out slightly, then bring them back to the center so they cross.

As you do this movement, make sure your legs are no higher than a 45-degree angle so that your abs keep you steady. Move slowly and steadily so the muscles work hard and you don't bob. Do not open your legs too far, just behind your hips.

You can vary this movement by lifting each leg a little higher while keeping the other leg slightly lowered so that you can do the scissoring movement up and down rather than left and right.

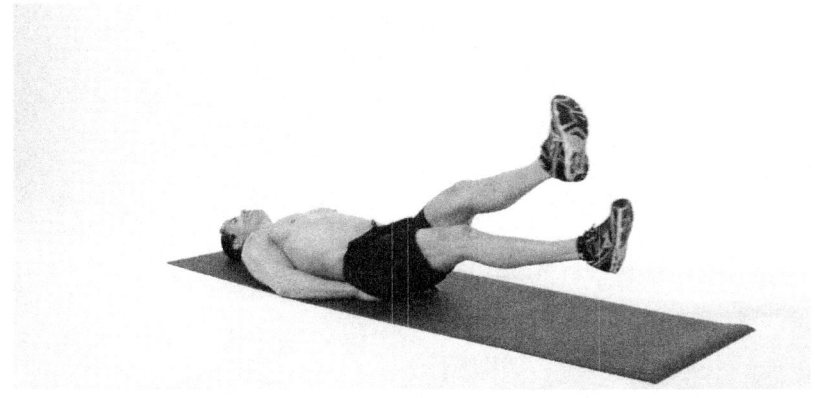

Tip 27: Side planks

Side planks are a little tricky, but very effective for your entire stomach, including your back.

    1. Lie on the mat with your arm under you.

    2. Lift up on your arm while lifting your legs so that only your arm and one foot are touching the mat. Keep your legs together. Your abs work very hard to support you in this position and you can hold it for a few seconds to get a good workout.

To add a challenge, use a free weight in your open hand and lift it right in front of you. Tighten your abs to keep them flexed and tense.

You can also lift the weight up in the air and aim it at the ceiling. This will challenge your balance and help tone and firm your center.

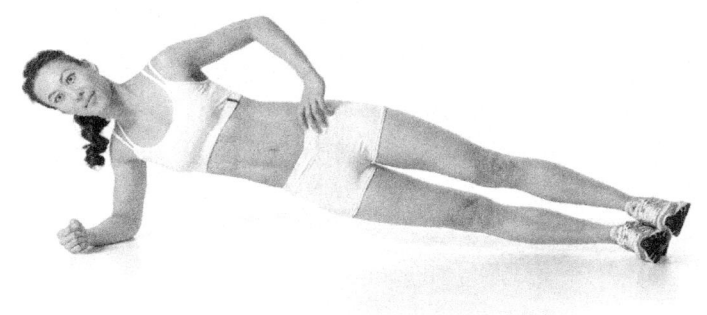

Tip 28: Forward bends

This exercise can help work the abs and straighten the back and hips, creating a lean and toned appearance and a strong midsection. The abs will support you as you move forward, but especially as you straighten up.

1. To make this simple but challenging move, stand with your feet a little wider than shoulder width apart,

arms stretched out to your sides so that your body forms a T-shape.

2. Next, twist around your waist and bend to the right so that your left hand is touching the floor that is just outside your right foot. Instead of bending your arms or knees, let the abs do all the work.

3. Stand up and repeat on the opposite side.

Pay close attention to your posture, because keeping your back straight ensures that the abdominal muscles do the work and you don't strain your back muscles.

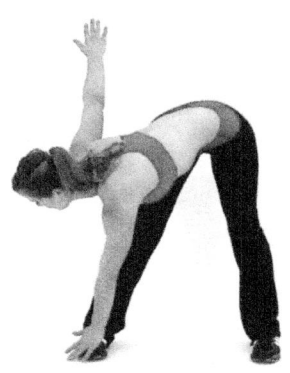

Tip 29: Rubber band training

Exercising with rubber bands can give you extra resistance so you can work your abs and get a lean look. Ribbons are easy to take with you when you are on the go and can be easily stowed away. So they are a great choice for keeping fit on the go and for those who live in an apartment or small house and don't have room for oversized equipment or free weights. For the most effective banded abs workout, choose one with the highest resistance.

1. Hook them onto a doorknob or something else that will keep you safe. Hold the straps when getting into position to do sit-ups or crunches, and pull on the straps as you move. This resistance that the ligaments offer will help tone the abs.

2. Go very slowly with the movement and do not turn too far, as you do not want to lose the resistance, but want to keep your abdominal muscles tense throughout to allow yourself a good workout.

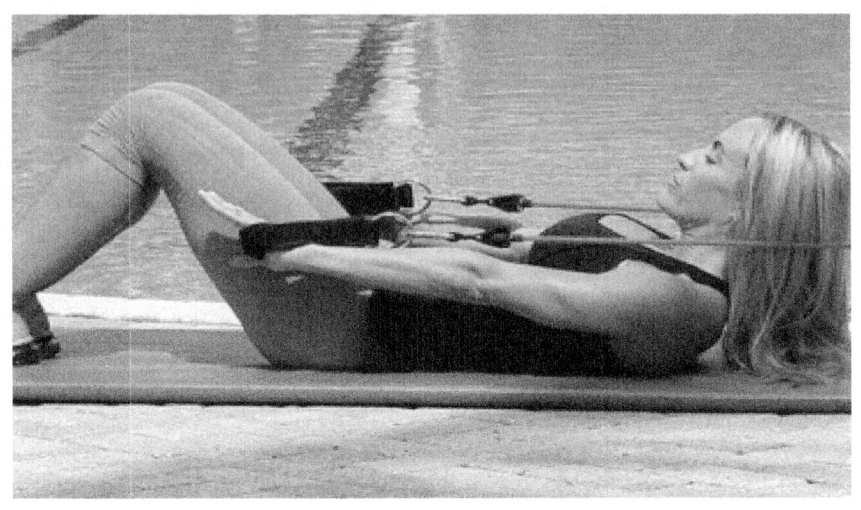

Tip 30: The hundred

The hundred is another popular Pilates exercise. You tone and tone your abs and abdominal area by making sure you can hold a position long enough. It might sound easy, but it's really very challenging.

1. Lie on your back with your legs raised at 45 degrees, arms by your sides.
2. Lift your torso forward, keeping it straight so your shoulders are just above the floor. You will feel your abs contract to maintain this position. Instead of lifting yourself so far that you lose resistance in your abs, just stay a few inches off the floor.

3. While staying in this position, just gently moving your arms up and down, do this a hundred times.

The arms shouldn't be much higher than the body as you are only supposed to keep your arms off the floor. If this exercise seems too challenging, put your legs up, knees bent, feet flat on the floor, as this will relieve pressure from the abdominal muscles. Gently roll your torso back onto the mat and rest before repeating the exercise!

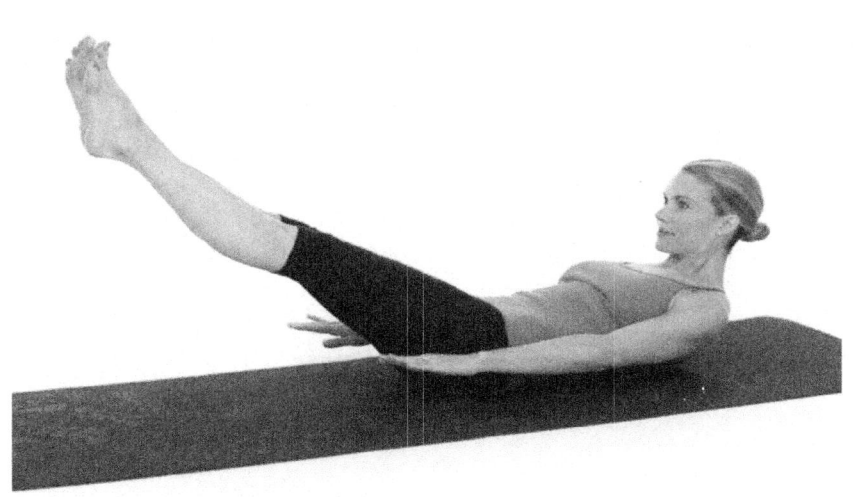

Tip 31: reverse sit-ups

For a very challenging workout for the abs, be sure to do the reverse sit-up. This movement causes your body to work very hard to keep you from falling backwards and it is a great exercise for burning fat and sculpting your core.

1. Start by sitting on your exercise mat with your legs in front of you, feet just slightly apart.
2. Cross your hands behind your head.
3. Sit back by bending at your hips, then continue moving backward until your torso is finally on the mat and you are fully reclined.
4. Instead of bending your back, keep your upper body straight. Your abs will work hard throughout the movement to keep you upright and balanced.
5. Since this movement works best when moving backwards rather than forward, you can get yourself back into a sitting position by pushing yourself up off the floor with your hands. Place your hands behind your head when you're ready to repeat the movement and move slowly so that you keep your abs moving.

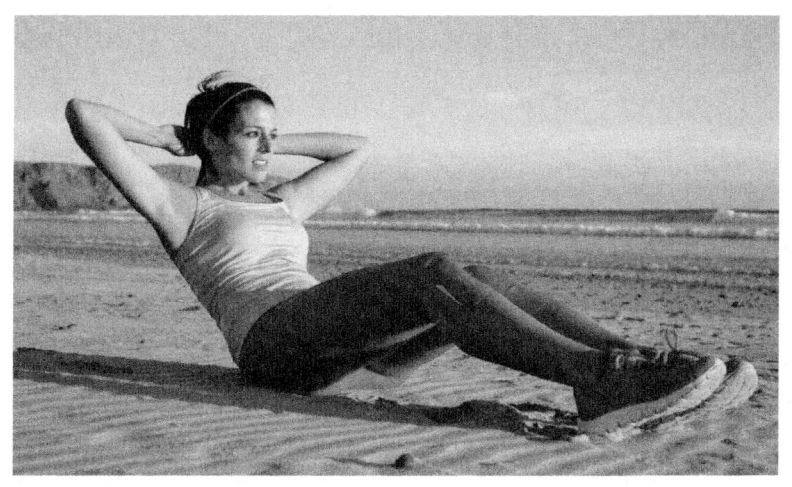

Conclusion

Now that you know the exercises you need to do to burn your belly fat and tone your belly and core. But none of this will do you any good if your diet is not right. In part of this book I have also explained to you what your diet should look like. But the best results to get, must you go on a diet or rather take on a new diet. In order to make this possible for you, we at the "Health & Fitness Acamedy" arranged a work with Cathrine Brahms. We are now giving you a book that will make you very successful. This book will you guarantee to your destination. You even get a third book with recipes to try out. If you enjoyed this book and want to share your positive thoughts, please could you take 30 seconds of your time and write me a review on Amazon. I appreciate your reviews because it helps me share my hard work! Thank you again and I wish you all the best!

Low carb breakfast recipes

Breakfast is considered the most important meal of the day, and of course it's important that you don't drive to work with your stomach growling. These recipes can be prepared quickly, and if you don't have much of an appetite in the morning, you can also take these dishes with you to work as a snack.

Crunchy cheese omelette

Calories: 248.1 kcal | Protein: 22.2 grams | Fat: 17.3 grams | Carbohydrates: 0.9 grams

Preparation time: 10 minutes

Ingredients for one serving:

1 tbsp Parmesan, finely grated | 2 eggs | 2 slices of Gouda cheese | Pepper | Rubbed thyme

Preparation:

1. Spread the parmesan in a coated pan without oil and let it melt slightly.

2. In the meantime, whisk the eggs and season with pepper and thyme.

3. Now slowly pour the seasoned eggs over the melted parmesan.

4. Now spread the Gouda on top and let the egg set.

5. Carefully fold the omelette with an ice spatula and let it stand for a minute without heat.

6. Arrange and sprinkle with fresh herbs as required.

7. You shouldn't need salt for the omelette as the parmesan and gouda are salty enough.

Creamy low carb scrambled eggs with smoked salmon

Calories: 285.7 kcal | Protein: 23.2 grams | Fat: 20.5 grams | Carbohydrates: 2.1 grams

Preparation time: 8 minutes

Ingredients for one serving:

2 eggs | 2 tbsp cream | Himalayan salt | Pepper | 1/2 teaspoon dill chopped | 50 grams of smoked salmon | some zest of an untreated organic lemon

Preparation:

1. Whisk the eggs with the cream and season sparingly with salt and pepper.
2. Process in a coated pan without fat to a scrambled egg that is not too dry.
3. Cut the salmon into strips and mix into the scrambled eggs.
4. Flavor with the zest of lemon and serve.
5. Sprinkle generously with dill before serving.
6. If you don't like dill that much, you can also use chives, parsley or coriander.

Savory low carb zucchini walnut muffins

Calories: 297.4 kcal | Protein: 52.1 grams | Fat: 41 grams | Carbohydrates: 12.5 grams

Preparation time: 23 minutes

Ingredients for 4 muffins:

2 eggs | 4 tbsp quark | 80 grams of almond flour | 1 pinch of baking soda | 4 tbsp chopped walnuts | 1 zucchini finely grated | Himalayan salt and pepper

Preparation:

1. Separate the eggs and use a whisk or hand mixer to beat the egg whites to a stiff snow.
2. Mix the egg yolks with the quark until smooth and season sparingly with salt and pepper.
3. Mix the almond flour with the baking soda, the chopped nuts and the finely grated zucchini and mix with the yolk.
4. Carefully fold in the egg whites and fill the batter into four baking tins.
5. The muffins are baked in the oven at 180 ° Celsius and using top and bottom heat for 15 minutes.

Oven eggs with oregano tomatoes

Calories: 204.6 kcal | Protein: 13.4 grams | Fat: 15.8 grams | Carbohydrates: 2.2 grams

Preparation time: 9 minutes

Ingredients for one serving:

2 eggs | 1 tomato | Fresh or dried oregano | Himalayan salt and pepper | 1/2 teaspoon olive oil

Preparation:

1. Cut the tomato into slices and layer in a small baking dish.
2. Season with salt, pepper and oregano and drizzle with the olive oil.

3. Beat the eggs over it and slide the casserole dish into the oven, which has been preheated to 200 ° Celsius.
4. Bake the eggs for 6 minutes on top and bottom heat and sprinkle with fresh herbs as required.

Low carb lime curd with fruits

Calories: 172.8 kcal | Protein: 17.5 grams | Fat: 6 grams | Carbohydrates: 12.2 grams

Preparation time: 6 minutes

Ingredients for one serving:

150 grams of cottage cheese | 2 tbsp cream | Juice and zest of half an untreated organic lime | 1 splash of sweetener or a little stevia | 20 grams of blackberries | 20 grams of raspberries | 20 grams of blueberries | some mint leaves or lemon balm to decorate

Preparation:

1. Mix the quark with the cream until smooth, flavor with the juice and zest of the lime and sweeten with the sweetener as required.
2. Pour into a bowl and cover with the berries.
3. Garnish with mint or lemon balm before enjoying.
4. You can also prepare the quark the evening before and store it in the refrigerator.

Chia pudding with strawberries

Calories: 150 kcal | Protein: 8.6 grams | Fat: 6.8 grams | Carbohydrates: 13.6 grams

Preparation time: 6 minutes - the pudding should however soak for a few hours

Ingredients for one serving:

150 grams of yogurt | 1 teaspoon xylitol or stevia | 1 tsp chia seeds | some fresh thyme leaves | 80 grams of strawberries

Preparation:

1. Mix the yoghurt with the sweetener and the chia seeds.
2. Flavor with the thyme and leave to soak in the refrigerator overnight.
3. Before serving, cut the strawberries into small pieces and fold in.
4. You can add a dash of lemon juice or a pinch of cinnamon to the chia pudding.

Matcha yogurt with mango

Calories: 145 kcal | Protein: 8.9 grams | Fat: 4.6 grams | Carbohydrates: 17 grams

Preparation time: 6 minutes

Ingredients for one serving:

130 grams of yogurt | 2 tbsp cream cheese | 1 level teaspoon matcha powder | some abrasion of an untreated organic lime | 1/2 mango

Preparation:

1. Stir the yoghurt with the cream cheese until smooth and work in the matcha powder with the whisk so that no lumps are formed.
2. Peel the mango and cut into small cubes.
3. Fold into the yoghurt along with the zest of the lime. You can easily prepare the yogurt the evening before, store it in the refrigerator and enjoy it for breakfast.

Low carb pancakes with berry sauce

Calories: 343.9 kcal | Protein: 33.8 grams | Fat: 17.9 grams | Carbohydrates: 11.9 grams

Preparation time: 13 minutes

Ingredients for one serving:

2 eggs | 80 ml low-fat milk | 3 tbsp almond flour | 1 pinch of Himalayan salt | 60 grams of fresh or frozen berry mix | 1 splash of liquid sweetener | 40 ml buttermilk

Preparation:

1. Whisk the eggs with the milk and stir with the almond flour until smooth.
2. Carefully season with a pinch of Himalayan salt.
3. Bake small pancakes from this thick batter in a non-fat non-stick pan.
4. Puree the berries with the buttermilk and sweeten with sweetener.
5. Serve the sauce with the pancakes.
6. You can easily puree the berries with a hand blender.

Grilled figs wrapped in bacon

Calories: 108.6 kcal | Protein: 6.2 grams | Fat: 3 grams | Carbohydrates: 14.2 grams

Preparation time: 6 minutes

Ingredients for one serving:

1 fig | 4 slices of raw ham such as Black Forest ham | some rosemary

Preparation:

1. Quarter the fig, season with finely chopped rosemary and wrap in the ham.
2. Fry crispy on all sides in a grill pan without fat.
3. The figs taste great not only for breakfast, but also as a small snack in between meals.

Spicy melon salad with crispy strips of bacon

Calories: 107.2 kcal | Protein: 6.4 grams | Fat: 6 grams | Carbohydrates: 6.9 grams

Preparation time: 10 minutes

Ingredients for one serving:

120 grams of honeydew melon | Juice and zest of half an untreated organic lime | 1 tbsp lemon balm finely chopped | freshly ground black pepper | 2 tbsp bacon diced

Preparation:

1. Cut the melon into 1 cm cubes and marinate with the juice and zest of the lime.
2. Mix in the lemon balm and ground pepper.
3. Fry the bacon in a non-fat frying pan until crispy, let it cool down briefly and mix it with the melon.
4. A slice of protein bread, which you can toast together with the bacon in the coated pan, tastes great with melon salad.

5. This way the bread absorbs the spicy aromas of the bacon.

Low carb cream cheese pancakes

Calories: 337.9 kcal | Protein: 32.8 grams | Fat: 20.3 grams | Carbohydrates: 6.6 grams

Preparation time: 11 minutes

Ingredients for one serving:

50 grams of cream cheese | 2 tbsp low-fat milk | 2 eggs | 4 tbsp almond flour or coconut flour | 1 pinch of baking powder | some vanilla flavor | 1 pinch of Himalayan salt | some sweetener, stevia or xylitol | 1 teaspoon butter

Preparation:
1. Mix the cream cheese with the milk until smooth.
2. Whisk and stir in the eggs.
3. Work in the almond flour and baking powder with the whisk and season with vanilla, salt and sweetener.
4. Bake the batter in a pan with melted, hot butter into small pancakes. Bake these on both sides for about 1.5 minutes until golden brown.

Strawberry curd with coconut

Calories: 298.8 kcal | Protein: 21.5 grams | Fat: 20.4 grams | Carbohydrates: 7.3 grams

Preparation time: 8 minutes

Ingredients for one serving:

100 grams of cottage cheese | 50 ml coconut milk | Juice of half an organic lime | some sweetener or stevia | 2 tbsp desiccated coconut, roasted | 60 grams of strawberries

Preparation:

1. Mix the quark with the coconut milk until smooth and season with lime juice and sweetener.
2. Cut the strawberries into small pieces and stir into the quark.
3. Place in a bowl and sprinkle with the roasted coconut flakes.
4. This quark can be prepared the day before and stored in the refrigerator.
5. You can also take the curd with you to work in a plastic box.

Spicy low carb avocado curd with bean sprouts

Calories: 168.5 kcal | Protein: 20.4 grams | Fat: 8.1 grams | Carbohydrates: 3.5 grams

Preparation time: 8 minutes

Ingredients for one serving:

1/4 avocado | 100 grams of cottage cheese | Himalayan salt and pepper | 1 squirt of lemon juice | 10 grams of bean sprouts

Preparation:

1. Peel the avocado and mash it with a fork.
2. Mix with the quark until smooth and season with salt, pepper and lemon juice.
3. Pour into a bowl and sprinkle with the sprouts.
4. You can easily grow various rungs yourself at home and use all the rungs of your choice.
5. Sprouts are great suppliers of vitamins and minerals, and they have next to no carbohydrates.

Fried eggs with melted tomatoes

Calories: 232.1 kcal | Protein: 13.6 grams | Fat: 18.5 grams | Carbohydrates: 2.8 grams

Preparation time: 10 minutes

Ingredients for one serving:

2 eggs | 1 tomato | 1 shallot | 2 tsp olive oil | 1/2 teaspoon rosemary finely chopped | Himalayan salt and pepper

Preparation:

1. Cut the tomato into six parts and roughly remove the seeds.
2. Dice the shallot and fry the tomato and shallot together with a teaspoon of olive oil over medium heat until translucent.
3. Season with the rosemary, salt and pepper and fry for 5 minutes.
4. Fry the eggs in the remaining olive oil to the fried eggs and serve with the tomatoes.
5. Enjoy a nice slice of protein bread with it.

Blood orange yogurt with chia seeds and lavender salt

Calories: 111 kcal | Protein: 5.8 grams | Fat: 5 grams | Carbohydrates: 10.7 grams

Preparation time: 6 minutes The chia seeds should soak for at least 1 hour

Ingredients for one serving:

1/2 blood orange filleted | 100 grams of yogurt | 1 tsp chia seeds | some sweetener, stevia or xylitol | 1 pinch of lavender salt

Preparation:

1. Puree the blood orange with the yoghurt and the chia seeds in a blender.
2. Season with sweetener and salt and leave to soak in the refrigerator for about an hour.
3. You can also easily prepare this yoghurt the evening before and store it in the refrigerator.

Light low carb recipes for a delicious lunch

The recipes for lunch can be cooked in next to no time, they taste absolutely delicious, are healthy and do not put a strain on the body. Lunch is often skipped, especially when working, because heavy dishes simply make you tired. After these lunches, however, you can continue with your usual daily routine, satisfied and energetic. Many of these dishes can also be conveniently taken to work and of course also taste absolutely good as dinner. Our dishes for morning, noon and evening should only give you a guideline, you can of course design the menu according to your mood. Make sure that your daily carbohydrate balance is always in the range of 30 grams.

Smoked trout fillet with fennel salad and wasabi dip

Calories: 239.3 kcal | Protein: 28.3 grams | Fat: 10.9 grams | Carbohydrates: 7 grams Preparation time: 10 minutes Ingredients for one serving: 120 grams of smoked trout | 1/2 tuber of fennel | 1 orange filleted | 1 pinch of cardamom | 1/2 teaspoon dill chopped | 1 tsp walnut oil | Himalayan salt and pepper | 2 tbsp sour cream | 1 splash of lime juice | 1/2 pinch of wasabi paste

Preparation:

1. Finely grate the fennel, cut the orange into pieces and mix with the fennel. Season with cardamom, dill, walnut oil, salt and pepper.

2. Mix the sour cream with the lime juice and the wasabi paste until smooth.

3. Depending on your own taste, you can use more or less wasabi.

4. Alternatively, horseradish can also be used for this.

5. Serve the trout with the salad and the dip and enjoy.

Fried eggs with fried poultry debreziner

Calories: 543.2 kcal | Protein: 27.8 grams | Fat: 47.1 grams | Carbohydrates: 2 grams Preparation time: 11 minutes Ingredients for one serving: 2 eggs | 2 tsp vegetable oil | Salt and pepper | 1 tbsp chives cut into rolls | 2 pieces of poultry Debreziner | 3 cherry tomatoes

Preparation:

1. Cut the tomatoes in half. Fry the eggs in a tablespoon of oil to make fried eggs.
2. Spread the cherry tomatoes in the pan, season with salt and pepper.
3. Slightly score the sausages with a knife and fry them all around in the remaining oil for about 3 minutes.
4. Arrange the fried eggs, sprinkle with chives and eat with the Debreziner sausages.
5. You can also use Wiener sausages or Frankfurter poultry sausages.
6. Make sure that the sausages are made without flour.

Creamed spinach with fried pumpkin

Calories: 292.6 kcal | Protein: 8.7 grams | Fat: 24.2 grams | Carbohydrates: 10.6 grams Preparation time: 23 minutes Ingredients for one serving: 80 grams of spinach leaves | 1/2 red onion | 1 clove of garlic | 1 teaspoon butter | 50 ml cream | 1 tbsp cottage cheese | Himalayan salt and pepper | some nutmeg grated | 80 grams of Hokkaido pumpkin | 1 teaspoon olive oil | 1/2 teaspoon rosemary chopped | 1 teaspoon of pumpkin seeds roasted and chopped

Preparation:

1. Chop the onion and garlic and sweat in butter until translucent.

2. Pour the cream on and stir in the cottage cheese.
3. Add the spinach leaves and simmer for 2 minutes.

4. Season with salt, pepper and nutmeg and remove from the heat.

5. Peel the pumpkin and cut into 1/2 cm thick pieces.

6. Fry these in olive oil until golden brown on all sides, season with salt, pepper and rosemary and serve with the spinach.

7. Sprinkle everything generously with the chopped and roasted pumpkin seeds.

8. You can also roast the pumpkin seeds yourself in a pan without oil.

9. This gives them a very intense aroma.

Spicy minute steaks with parmesan egg

Calories: 346 kcal | Protein: 39.8 grams | Fat: 20.4 grams | Carbohydrates: 0.8 grams Preparation time: 12 minutes Ingredients for one serving: 140 grams of minute steaks, (pork, beef or poultry) | 1/2 teaspoon olive oil | 1/2 teaspoon curry paste red from the Asia store | 1 egg | 1 tbsp parmesan, finely grated

Preparation:

1. Mix the olive oil with the red curry paste well and brush the meat well with it.

2. Now fry the meat in a grill pan without fat over high heat on both sides for one minute each.

3. Fry a fried egg in a non-stick pan, sprinkle with parmesan and serve with the meat.

4. A small leaf salad with a dressing of yogurt and lemon juice goes perfectly with the minute steaks.

Greek stir-fry with raw lamb ham

Calories: 297.9 kcal | Protein: 17.5 grams | Fat: 21.5 grams | Carbohydrates: 8.9 grams Preparation time: 20 minutes Ingredients for one serving: 1/2 zucchini | 1/4 yellow pepper | 1/4 red pepper | 1/4 eggplant | 1/2 red onion | 2 tomatoes | 1 tbsp olive oil | Thyme | Himalayan salt and pepper | 50 grams of sheep's cheese, firm | 30 grams of lamb ham thinly sliced

Preparation:

1. Cut the zucchini, bell pepper, aubergine, onion and tomato into 1 cm cubes.
2. Roast them together in the olive oil for about 10 minutes.
3. Stir constantly so that the vegetables don't get too dark.
4. Season to taste with salt and pepper and flavor with thyme.
5. Arrange on a plate and crumble the sheep's cheese over it.
6. Drape the lamb ham over it.
7. Instead of lamb ham, you can also use Bündnerfleisch or prosciutto.

Stuffed zucchini Tuscany Art

Calories: 149.5 kcal | Protein: 7 grams | Fat: 5.5 grams | Carbohydrates: 18 grams Preparation time: 23 minutes Ingredients for one serving: 1 zucchini | 1 shallot | 60 grams of cherry tomatoes | 1 fig | 1/2 pear | 8 black or green olives | Himalayan salt and pepper | Fresh or dried basil | 2 tbsp parmesan

Preparation:

1. Cut the zucchini lengthways and carefully scrape out the core with a spoon.
2. Chop the shallot, cherry tomatoes, fig and pear and mix together.
3. Season with salt and pepper and fill the zucchini with it.
4. Lightly press the olives into the filling and sprinkle with the basil.
5. Finally, spread the parmesan on top and place the zucchini on a baking sheet lined with baking paper.
6. Bake in the oven at 200 ° Celsius for 15 minutes with top and bottom heat.

Pasta salad with konjac noodles

Calories: 318 kcal | Protein: 19.6 grams | Fat: 21.2 grams | Carbohydrates: 12.2 grams Preparation time: 15 minutes Ingredients for one serving: 50 grams of konjac noodles | 1/4 green pepper | 1/2 yellow pepper | 1/2 apple red | 1/2 cucumber | 20 grams of turkey ham diced | 1 tbsp walnuts chopped | 20 grams of sliced cheese, diced | 1/2 chicory red | Juice and zest of half an untreated organic lemon | 1 tbsp sour cream | Himalayan salt and pepper | 1 tbsp chives chopped | 1 teaspoon chervil chopped

Preparation:

1. Rinse the konjac noodles and cook or blanch briefly according to the instructions on the packet.

2. Rinse with cold water and set aside.

3. Mix the juice and zest of the lemon with the sour cream and mix with the chives and chervil.

4. Salt and pepper well.

5. Finely dice the paprika, coarsely grate the apple and cucumber, cut the chicory into strips and stir everything together with the diced turkey ham.

6. Mix in the walnuts and also mix in the cheese.

7. Fold in the konjac noodles and add the prepared marinade.

8. Season briefly as needed and enjoy.

Turkey steak with herb and cream cheese sauce

Calories: 231.6 kcal | Protein: 36.9 grams | Fat: 7.2 grams | Carbohydrates: 4.8 grams Preparation time: 16 minutes Ingredients for one serving: 150 grams of turkey steak | 1 shallot | 1 clove of garlic | 1 teaspoon butter | 1 tbsp lemon juice | 80 ml of broth | 1 tbsp cream cheese | 1/2 teaspoon chopped parsley | 1/2 teaspoon chopped tarragon | 1/2 teaspoon chopped coriander | Himalayan salt | White pepper

Preparation:

1. Salt and pepper the meat and grill in a grill pan without fat on both sides for two minutes each.

2. Cut the shallot and the garlic into small pieces and sauté them together in the butter.

3. Deglaze with the lemon juice and immediately add the broth.

4. Bring to the boil briefly and stir in the cream cheese with a whisk.

5. Remove the sauce from the heat and stir in the herbs.

6. Season to taste with salt and pepper, briefly put the meat in the sauce, let it stand for a minute, serve and feast.

Chicken curry with papaya and mango

Calories: 317 kcal | Protein: 42.9 grams | Fat: 10.2 grams | Carbohydrates: 13.4 grams Preparation time: 14 minutes Ingredients for one serving: 130 grams of skinless chicken breast | 1/2 red onion | 1 tbsp vegetable oil | 1/2 teaspoon curry powder yellow | Juice of half a lime | 1/2 stick of celery | 1/2 mango | 50 grams of papaya | 80 ml of broth | 3 tbsp yogurt | 1 red chilli | some Himalayan salt | 1 tbsp chopped coriander

Preparation:

1. Cut the chicken into thin strips and finely dice the onion.

2. Sear both together in the oil for two minutes.

3. Sprinkle with the curry powder and let the curry roast briefly.

4. Deglaze with the lime juice and immediately add the stock.

5. Cut the celery, mango and papaya into 1 cm cubes and add to the pan as well.

6. Chop the chilli or use a mortar and mix with the yoghurt.

7. Now stir the hot yoghurt into the broth and season gently with salt.

8. Sprinkle the dish generously with chopped coriander before serving.

9. You can also use parsley instead of coriander and replace the chilli with a little pepper if you like it milder.

Chicken breast with paprika strips

Calories: 263.1 kcal | Protein: 47.1 grams | Fat: 5.1 grams | Carbohydrates: 7.2 grams Preparation time: 22 minutes Ingredients for one serving: 140 grams of skinless chicken breast | Himalayan salt and pepper | Mild paprika powder | 1/4 red pepper | 1/4 yellow pepper | 1/4 green pepper | 1/2 red onion | 1 tbsp cream cheese | 2 sprigs of thyme

Preparation:

1. Cut the chicken breast into three equal pieces and rub salt, pepper and paprika.

2. Cut the bell pepper and onion into strips, mix everything together and place in a small baking dish.

3. Salt, pepper and flavor with thyme.

4. Place the chicken breast on top and spread the cream cheese over it.

5. Now put it in the oven preheated to 180 ° Celsius and bake for 15 minutes with a fan oven.

6. Take out of the oven, arrange on a plate and enjoy.

Pollack in a curry broth with cherry tomatoes

Calories: 289.8 kcal | Protein: 27.9 grams | Fat: 17.5 grams | Carbohydrates: 5.4 grams Preparation time: 18 minutes Ingredients for one serving: 130 grams of pollack filleted | 1 shallot | 1 clove of garlic | 1/2 teaspoon vegetable oil | 1/2 teaspoon curry powder yellow | 2 allspice grains | 2 cloves | 2 cardamom pods | 1 stick of celery | 1 tomato | 500 ml broth | 2 spring onions | Himalayan salt and pepper

Preparation:

1. Finely chop the shallot and the clove of garlic and lightly toast them together with the curry powder in the oil.
2. Add the allspice, cloves and cardamom and pour the broth on top.
3. Let it boil briefly once.
4. Cut the celery and tomatoes into small pieces and add them to the stock with the whole fish.
5. Season with salt and pepper and simmer over medium heat for 12 minutes.
6. Cut the spring onion into small pieces.
7. Remove the fish and vegetables from the broth, serve with a little liquid and sprinkle with spring onions.
8. Store the rest of the brew in the refrigerator or freeze it.

Baked camembert with bacon

Calories: 708.6 kcal | Protein: 56.5 grams | Fat: 51.8 grams | Carbohydrates: 4.8 grams Preparation time: 12 minutes Ingredients for one serving: 1 Camembert with about 125 grams | 6 thin slices of pork belly or bacon | 1 pinch of hot paprika powder | 1 tbsp almond flour | 1 egg | 2 tbsp low-fat milk | 4 tbsp finely grated almonds | 1 teaspoon chopped rosemary

Preparation:

1. Rub the camembert with the paprika and evenly wrap the bacon.
2. Roll in the almond flour.
3. Whisk the egg with the low-fat milk and pull the cheese through.
4. Mix the grated almonds with the rosemary and bread the camembert in it. Pull the cheese through the egg one more time and bread it again.
5. Place on the grill rack and heat the oven to 200 ° Celsius.
6. Bake the camembert for about 7 minutes in the fan oven. You can also prepare the Camembert in the air fryer.

Frittata with smoked salmon and dill

Calories: 442.9 kcal | Protein: 40.3 grams | Fat: 29.7 grams | Carbohydrates: 3.6 grams Preparation time: 20 minutes Ingredients for one serving: 2 eggs | 60 ml buttermilk | 100 grams of smoked salmon | Juice and zest of half an untreated organic lemon | Himalayan salt and pepper | 1 tbsp dill chopped | 20 grams of butter cheese grated

Preparation:

1. Whisk the eggs with the buttermilk and season with the juice and zest of the lemon, with salt, pepper and dill.
2. Pour into a round tart pan and spread the coarsely chopped smoked salmon on top.
3. Sprinkle with the butter cheese and heat the oven to 190 ° Celsius.
4. Bake the frittata on top and bottom heat for 15 minutes.
5. A small mixed salad that you can marinate with a little apple cider vinegar and olive oil tastes great with it.

Sausage salad with radishes, chilli and coriander

Calories: 191.1 kcal | Protein: 10.8 grams | Fat: 7.9 grams | Carbohydrates: 19.2 grams Preparation time: 10 minutes Ingredients for one serving: 100 grams of poultry sausage | 3 radishes | 2 gherkins with no added sugar | 1 red chilli | 1/4 red pepper | 1/2 chicory | 1/2 bunch of coriander chopped | 1 tomato | Himalayan salt | 2 tbsp apple cider vinegar | 4 tbsp water or broth | 1 tbsp vegetable oil

Preparation:

1. Cut the poultry sausage into thin strips, cut the radishes and pickles into slices, and dice the chilli, paprika, chicory and tomato.

2. Mix everything together with the chopped coriander.

3. Mix apple cider vinegar, water and oil into a marinade, lightly salt and use it to dress the sausage salad.

Vegetable thalers baked with bacon and cheese

Calories: 390.1 kcal | Protein: 23.3 grams | Fat: 27.7 grams | Carbohydrates: 11.9 grams Preparation time: 20 minutes Ingredients for one serving: 1/2 zucchini | 1/4 carrot | 20 grams of celeriac | 1 teaspoon sesame seeds | 1 egg | 2 tbsp oat bran | 1 tbsp grated almonds | 1 teaspoon parsley chopped | Himalayan salt and pepper | 1/2 teaspoon lovage chopped | 20 grams of bacon diced | 2 tbsp grated mountain cheese | some marjoram

Preparation:

1. Grate the zucchini, carrot and celery very finely.
2. Mix with the sesame, egg, oat bran and almonds.
3. Mix in the parsley and lovage and season with salt and pepper.
4. Shape this mass with wet hands and fry in a non-stick pan for 2 minutes on each side.
5. Mix the bacon with mountain cheese and marjoram.
6. Cover the thalers with it and place them on a baking sheet lined with baking paper.
7. If the grill function is used, grill for about 3 minutes.

Chicken Caprese

Calories: 368.9 kcal | Protein: 52.1 grams | Fat: 16.5 grams | Carbohydrates: 3 grams Preparation time: 20

minutes Ingredients for one serving: 130 grams of skinless chicken breast | 1 tbsp olive oil | some zest of an untreated organic lemon | 1/2 bunch of basil | Himalayan salt and pepper | 1/2 tomato | 1/2 scoop of mozzarella

Preparation:

1. Salt and pepper the chicken.

2. Process the olive oil with the lemon zest and the basil in a blender into a pesto.

3. Salt and pepper and brush the chicken breast with it.

4. Make a deep cut in the top of the chicken breast and cut the tomato and mozzarella into slices.

5. Now insert the tomato and mozzarella into the notches on the chicken.

6. Place on a baking sheet lined with baking paper and cook at 180 ° Celsius for 12 minutes on top and bottom heat.

Baked ham and cheese rolls with asparagus

Calories: 560 kcal | Protein: 37.3 grams | Fat: 38.4 grams | Carbohydrates: 16.3 grams Preparation time: 16 minutes Ingredients for one serving: 8 slices of turkey ham | 4 slices of Gouda cheese | 2 stalks of green asparagus | 1 tbsp almond flour | 1 tbsp low-fat milk | 2 tbsp walnuts finely grated | Himalayan salt and pepper | 1 tbsp sour cream | 1/2 teaspoon mustard with no added sugar

Preparation:

1. Place two slices of ham next to each other, overlapping, and top with a slice of cheese.
2. Halve the asparagus and place on top of the cheese.
3. Roll up the ham and toss in the almond flour.
4. Whisk the egg with the milk and pull the rolls through.
5. Bread in the walnuts and place on a baking sheet lined with baking paper.
6. Bake the rolls for 6 minutes at 180 ° Celsius and convection.
7. Mix the sour cream, mustard, salt and pepper into a dip and serve with the rolls.
8. You can also prepare the rolls in the Airfryer.

Fast low carb main courses

These low carb recipes are suitable for quick dinners so that you don't have to reach for ready-made products and fast food after a long day at work. You will love these recipes and be surprised how quickly these delicacies can be cooked.

Low carb gourmet fillet of saithe

Calories: 319.1 kcal | Protein: 29.9 grams | Fat: 20.3 grams | Carbohydrates: 4.2 grams Preparation time: 25 minutes Ingredients for one serving: 140 grams of pollack fillet | Himalayan salt | white pepper | Lemon juice | 1 tbsp butter | 1 teaspoon dill chopped | 1 teaspoon chives in rolls | 2 tbsp grated almonds | 1 pinch of mustard medium hot without added sugar

Preparation:

1. Salt and pepper the fish and drizzle with lemon juice.
2. Knead the butter with the dill, chives, almonds and mustard and spread on the fish.
3. Place in a small baking dish and heat the oven to 180 ° Celsius.
4. Cook the fish on top and bottom heat for 15 minutes.
5. Take out of the oven and enjoy with a small mixed salad.

Zucchini Spaghetti with Prawns and Garlic

Calories: 159.7 kcal | Protein: 21.8 grams | Fat: 5.7 grams | Carbohydrates: 5.3 grams Preparation time: 12 minutes Ingredients for one serving: 1 zucchini | 1/2 red onion | 2 cloves of garlic | 1 tbsp butter | 100 grams of shrimp without shell | 1/2 red pepper | Juice of half a lemon | Himalayan salt | Pepper | 1/2 tbsp coriander chopped | 1/2 teaspoon rosemary finely chopped

Preparation:

1. Use the vegetable peeler to process the zucchini into fine noodles.

2. Chop the onion and garlic and cut the bell pepper into strips.

3. Heat the butter in a pan and fry the prawns with onion, garlic and paprika for 2 minutes.

4. Add the zucchini noodles and toss with the rosemary and coriander.

5. Deglaze with the lemon juice and season with salt and pepper.

6. Steam for about 2 minutes over medium heat and serve.

7. If necessary, you can refine the "noodles" with a little grated Parmesan.

Italian low carb burger

Calories: 297.5 kcal | Protein: 36 grams | Fat: 15.1 grams | Carbohydrates: 4.4 grams Preparation time: 15 minutes Ingredients for one serving: 150 grams of ground beef | 1/2 onion | 1 clove of garlic | 1/2 teaspoon hot mustard with no added sugar | rubbed some thyme | 1 pinch of ground caraway seeds | 1 tomato | 1/2 scoop of mozzarella | 8 basil leaves | salt and pepper

Preparation:

1. Finely chop the onion and garlic and knead with the meat and mustard.

2. Season lightly with salt and pepper and season with thyme and caraway seeds.

3. Shape into two patties with wet hands and fry in a non-oiled pan on all sides for 2 minutes.

4. The patties are used as "burger bread".

5. Cut the tomato and mozzarella into slices and layer them with the basil between the meat loaves.

6. Place on a baking sheet lined with baking paper and bake in the oven at 200 ° for 3 minutes.

Chicken Szeged goulash

Calories: 331.8 kcal | Protein: 38.9 grams | Fat: 17.8 grams | Carbohydrates: 4 grams Preparation time: 25 minutes Ingredients for one serving: 120 grams of chicken thighs loosened | 1/2 onion | 1 clove of garlic | 1 teaspoon tomato paste with no added sugar | 1/2 teaspoon mild paprika | 1 pinch of hot pepper | Dried thyme | Dried marjoram | Cumin | 150 ml chicken broth | 50 grams of sauerkraut with no added sugar | Salt | Pepper | 1 tbsp vegetable oil | 1 tbsp creme fraiche

Preparation:

1. Cut the chicken into 1 cm cubes, chop the onion and garlic and fry them together in the vegetable oil for a good 3 minutes.

2. Add the tomato paste and roast for 2 minutes.

3. Add paprika, thyme and marjoram and roast briefly.

4. Pour the chicken stock and simmer for 12 minutes.

5. Add the sauerkraut and season with salt, pepper and cumin.

6. After simmering for 5 minutes, arrange over medium heat and garnish with the creme fraiche before serving.

Monkfish skewer on tomato and spring onion lettuce

Calories: 216.2 kcal | Protein: 25.3 grams | Fat: 11.8 grams | Carbohydrates: 2.2 grams Preparation time: 12 minutes Ingredients for one serving: 150 grams of angler fish fillet | 2 slices of bacon | Himalayan salt | Steak pepper | some lime juice | 1 stick of lemongrass | 3 spring onions with green | 40 grams of cherry tomatoes yellow | 40 cherry tomatoes red | 1/2 bunch of chervil chopped | 1 tbsp apple cider vinegar | 1 tbsp olive oil | 1 dash of sweetener

Preparation:

1. Salt, pepper and sour the fish with lime juice and cut into 3 equal pieces.
2. Skewer alternately with the bacon on the lemongrass.
3. Fry well on all sides in a grill pan without fat for 4 minutes each.
4. Cut the spring onion into rings, halve the cherry tomatoes and mix with the spring onion and chervil.
5. Marinate with a dressing of apple cider vinegar, olive oil and sweetener and serve with the skewer.
6. If you don't have lemongrass, you can use ordinary wooden skewers.
7. The lemongrass only provides a special, additional aroma.

Stuffed turkey schnitzel with cheese, onion and chilli

Calories: 280 kcal | Protein: 40.7 grams | Fat: 12 grams | Carbohydrates: 2.3 grams Preparation time: 17 minutes Ingredients for one serving: 140 grams of turkey schnitzel | Salt and pepper | 20 grams of grated Emmental cheese | 1/2 red onion | 1 red chilli | 2 sage leaves | 1 tbsp mountain cheese grated

Preparation:

1. Pound the turkey thinly and season with salt and pepper.
2. Cut the onion and the chilli into slices and mix with the chopped sage and Emmentaler.
3. Spread on the schnitzel and fold in the meat.
4. Fix with a toothpick. Place on a baking sheet lined with baking paper and sprinkle with the mountain cheese.
5. Heat the oven to 170 ° Celsius and cook the turkey on top and bottom heat for 12 minutes.
6. The meat also tastes wonderful when cut into strips cold as a snack.

Prawns with black sesame seeds on arugula

Calories: 350.9 kcal | Protein: 31.7 grams | Fat: 21.3 grams | Carbohydrates: 8.1 grams Preparation time: 11 minutes Ingredients for one serving: 140 grams of shrimp without shell and cleaned | 1 tbsp sesame oil | 1 tbsp black sesame seeds | Juice and zest of an untreated organic lime | Himalayan salt | Pepper | 50 grams of arugula | 1 tbsp roasted pine nuts | 1/4 yellow pepper | 2 date tomatoes | 1 teaspoon raspberry vinegar | 2 tbsp water | 1 tbsp walnut oil | 40 grams of fresh or frozen raspberries

Preparation:

1. Fry the prawns in the sesame oil for 2 minutes until translucent and sprinkle with the sesame seeds.

2. Season with salt, pepper, lime juice and zest.
3. Mix the raspberry vinegar with water and walnut oil and season with salt and pepper.
4. Cut the peppers into cubes and the tomatoes into slices.
5. Mix both with the rocket and fold in the pine nuts and raspberries.
6. Marinate with the dressing and serve with the prawns.
7. A slice of toasted egg white bread goes perfectly with this dish.
8. Packed in a plastic can, you can also take this food with you to work, as the prawns taste wonderfully aromatic even when cold.

Fillet of beef with fried watermelon

Calories: 319.3 kcal | Protein: 34.8 grams | Fat: 16.5 grams | Carbohydrates: 7.9 grams Preparation time: 10 minutes Ingredients for one serving: 180 grams of beef fillet | Fleur de Sel | colored pepper | 1 sprig of rosemary | 2 sprigs of thyme | 2 cloves of garlic | 1 tbsp olive oil | 100 grams of watermelon seedless

Preparation:

1. Salt and pepper the meat and fry in olive oil with rosemary, thyme and garlic.

2. Fry the meat for about 3 minutes on each side.
3. As soon as you turn the meat, add the watermelon to the pan and roast it with it.
4. Arrange everything together and add a little salt and pepper if necessary.

Pork fillet with paprika gorgonzola sauce

Calories: 232.4 kcal | Protein: 37.6 grams | Fat: 7.6 grams | Carbohydrates: 3.4 grams Preparation time: 12 minutes Ingredients for one serving: 150 grams of pork tenderloin | 1 tbsp olive oil | 1 shallot | 1/2 red pepper | 1/2 teaspoon sweet paprika | 1 tbsp apple cider vinegar | 1 pinch of ginger powder | 80 ml of broth | 10 grams of Gorgonzola or blue cheese of your choice | 1 tbsp chives in rolls | salt and pepper

Preparation:

1. Divide the pork tenderloin into three medallions of the same size and flatten them lightly with your hand.

2. Salt and pepper the meat and brush with the paprika powder.
3. Cut the shallot and bell pepper into strips.
4. Fry the meat in the olive oil on both sides for 2 minutes each, remove from the pan and keep warm.

5. Roast the shallot and paprika in the same and deglaze with apple cider vinegar.

6. Season with ginger and add the broth.

7. Bring to the boil briefly and crumble the Gorgonzola.

8. Let the cheese melt over medium heat, stirring constantly.

9. Put the meat back in the pan, swirl briefly and serve.

10. Sprinkle with chives or herbs of your choice before serving.

Minced meat pan with basil

Calories: 333.4 kcal | Protein: 44.2 grams | Fat: 14.6 grams | Carbohydrates: 6.3 grams Preparation time: 18 minutes Ingredients for one serving: 130 grams of minced poultry | 1/2 onion | 1/2 teaspoon curry paste red from the Asia store | Juice of half a lime | 1/2 stick of celery | 50 ml coconut milk | 1 pinch of xylitol or a splash of sweetener | Soy sauce | Fish sauce | 8 basil leaves | 1 dried chilli pepper | 2 tbsp hazelnuts chopped | 50 ml broth | 1 teaspoon coconut oil

Preparation:

1. Dice the onion and fry it with the minced meat in coconut oil.

2. Add the curry paste and roast for a few minutes.

3. Cut the celery into small pieces and add to the pan.

4. Season with lime juice, soy sauce and fish sauce.

5. Add the whole dried chilli and the hazelnuts and season with sweetener.

6. Deglaze with the stock and pour on the coconut milk.

7. Let it simmer for 5 minutes over medium heat, add seasoning as required and serve.

Chicken schnitzel in a parmesan egg shell

Calories: 459.4 kcal | Protein: 58.3 grams | Fat: 24.6 grams | Carbohydrates: 1.2 grams Preparation time: 10 minutes Ingredients for one serving: 140 grams of chicken schnitzel | Salt and pepper | 2 sage leaves | 1 tbsp almond flour | 1 egg | 3 teaspoons of parmesan, finely grated | 1 teaspoon vegetable oil | 1 teaspoon butter

Preparation:

1. Pound the schnitzel thinly, season with salt and pepper and press the sage well onto the meat.

2. Now roll the meat well in the flour.

3. Whisk the egg and mix with the parmesan.

4. Pull the schnitzel through and wet all over with egg.

5. Heat the vegetable oil together with the butter in a pan and bake the schnitzel in it until golden brown.

6. You can also prepare the schnitzel in the Airfryer.

7. Line the cooking basket with baking paper and bake the schnitzel at 180 ° Celsius for 10 minutes.

Baked salmon with broccoli and cauliflower

Calories: 460.7 kcal | Protein: 32.4 grams | Fat: 32.7 grams | Carbohydrates: 9.2 grams Preparation time: 15

minutes Ingredients for one serving: 130 grams of skinless salmon fillet | 50 grams of broccoli | 50 grams of cauliflower | 100 ml cream | 2 tbsp cream cheese | 1 tbsp lovage chopped (Maggi herb) | Juice of half a lemon | Salt and pepper | 1 tbsp roasted almond flakes

Preparation:

1. Salt and pepper the fish and place in a small baking dish.
2. Cut the broccoli and cauliflower into small florets and drape around the fish.
3. Mix the cream cheese with the lovage and lemon juice and season with salt and pepper.
4. Spread over the fish and sprinkle with flaked almonds.
5. Heat the oven to 180 ° Celsius and cook the fish in a fan oven for 12 minutes.

Saddle of pork steak with pumpkin crust

Calories: 452.5 kcal | Protein: 44.3 grams | Fat: 25.7 grams | Carbohydrates: 11 grams Preparation time: 18 minutes Ingredients for one serving: 160 grams of pork loin steak without rind | Salt and pepper | 50 grams of pumpkin | 1 tbsp chopped pumpkin seeds | 1 egg yolk | some dried marjoram | 2 tbsp oat bran | 1/2 teaspoon horseradish freshly torn

Preparation:

1. Salt and pepper the meat and fry in a grill pan without fat on both sides for 2 minutes each.

2. Finely grate the pumpkin and mix it with the chopped pumpkin seeds, egg yolk, marjoram, oat bran and horseradish.

3. Lightly salt and pepper.

4. Cover the meat with it and place on a parchment-lined baking sheet.

5. Heat the oven to 170 ° Celsius and bake the meat for 12 minutes on top and bottom heat.

Chicken in mushroom sauce

Calories: 238.8 kcal | Protein: 42 grams | Fat: 6.4 grams | Carbohydrates: 3.3 grams Preparation time: 15 minutes Ingredients for one serving: 120 grams of skinless chicken breast | 4 mushrooms | 3 small shallots | 1/4 yellow carrot | 120 ml chicken broth | 2 tbsp sour cream | some thyme fresh or dried | 1 teaspoon parsley chopped | Salt and pepper | 1 squirt of lemon juice

Preparation:

1. Cut the chicken into thin strips and quarter the mushrooms.

2. Cut the carrot into small cubes.

3. Bring the broth to a boil and add the meat, mushrooms, sliced shallots and diced carrots.

4. Let it cook for 10 minutes and then stir in the sour cream.

5. Season with thyme and season with salt, pepper and lemon juice.

6. Simmer for another 2 minutes over medium heat and sprinkle with parsley before serving.

Pikeperch with almond spinach

Calories: 365 kcal | Protein: 32.5 grams | Fat: 22.6 grams | Carbohydrates: 7.9 grams Preparation time: 12 minutes Ingredients for one serving: 150 grams of pikeperch fillet | 80 grams of spinach leaves | 1/2 onion | 1 clove of garlic | 1 pinch of baking soda | 2 tbsp almonds chopped | 60 ml cream | Salt and pepper | ground some nutmeg | some lemon juice | 2 teaspoons of butter

Preparation:

1. Salt and pepper the fish and sour with the lemon juice.

2. Fry skin-side down in a teaspoon of butter.

3. Fry on the skin side for 3 minutes, remove from the heat, turn and let steep for 2 minutes.

4. Cut the onion and garlic into small pieces and sweat together with the chopped almonds in the remaining butter until translucent.

5. Roughly chop the spinach leaves and add.

6. Pour the cream on and add baking soda.

7. Season with salt, pepper and nutmeg.

8. Simmer for a minute and serve with the pikeperch.

9. You can of course use any fish of your choice.

10. Cod, perch, and haddock also work well with this dish.

Veal schnitzel au gratin with sheep's cheese and bacon

Calories: 558 kcal | Protein: 39.9 grams | Fat: 43.6 grams | Carbohydrates: 1.6 grams Preparation time: 14 minutes Ingredients for one serving: 140 grams of veal escalope | 1 tbsp almond flour | Salt and pepper | 1 tbsp butter | 1 tbsp bacon diced | 30 grams goat cheese soft | 1 teaspoon walnuts chopped | 1 tbsp parsley chopped | 60 ml vegetable stock

Preparation:

1. Beat the schnitzel thinly, season with salt and pepper and fry in butter on both sides for one minute each.

2. Remove from the pan and stir the almond flour into the remaining butter.

3. Pour in the broth.

4. Stir with the whisk, bring to the boil once and set aside.

5. Place the schnitzel on a baking tray lined with baking paper and mix the bacon cubes with goat cheese, walnuts and parsley.

6. Spread on the meat and bake at 180 ° Celsius and top and bottom heat for 8 minutes.

7. Arrange on a plate, pour the sauce over them and enjoy.

Venison fillet on oven pumpkin

Calories: 366.7 kcal | Protein: 33.4 grams | Fat: 24.7 grams | Carbohydrates: 2.7 grams Preparation time: 18 minutes Ingredients for one serving: 140 grams of venison fillet | Salt and pepper | 1 tbsp olive oil | 1/2 teaspoon parsley chopped | 1/2 teaspoon chervil chopped | 1/2 teaspoon rosemary finely chopped | 1 teaspoon hazelnuts chopped | 80 grams of Hokkaido pumpkin | some thyme | 1 pinch of paprika powder mild | 1 pinch of cinnamon

Preparation:

1. Salt and pepper the meat and fry in the olive oil on all sides for about 3 minutes.
2. Mix the parsley, chervil, rosemary and hazelnuts and roll the meat in them.
3. Press the breading well with your hands.
4. Place on a baking tray lined with baking paper.
5. Cut the pumpkin into slices about 0.5 cm thick and season with thyme, paprika, cinnamon, salt and pepper.
6. Also place on the baking sheet and cook everything together at 160 ° Celsius with upper and lower heat for 15 minutes.

Creamy mince pan with mushrooms

Calories: 355.5 kcal | Protein: 30.1 grams | Fat: 21.9 grams | Carbohydrates: 9.5 grams Preparation time: 14 minutes Ingredients for one serving: 130 grams of minced beef, lean | 1/2 onion | 50 grams of chanterelles | 50 grams of king oyster mushrooms | 1/4 pear | 2 tbsp apple cider vinegar | 100 ml vegetable stock | 50 ml cream | Salt and pepper | dried marjoram | 1 tbsp chives in rolls | 1 teaspoon olive oil

Preparation:

1. Chop the onion and fry it with the minced meat in the olive oil.

2. Cut the chanterelles and mushrooms into bite-sized pieces and add them to the pan as well.
3. Dice the pear, add, toss and deglaze with apple cider vinegar.
4. Pour in the broth and season with salt, pepper and marjoram.
5. Simmer for about 8 minutes.
6. Refine with the cream, let simmer briefly, arrange and sprinkle with chives before serving.

Low carb snacks and side dishes

These low carb recipes are great for a small snack in between. The small dishes are also ideal as side dishes for lunch and dinner. When combining snacks and side dishes, always pay attention to the total daily turnover of carbohydrates. Calories and fat are negligible in a low carb diet - this means that you are guaranteed not to go hungry and still lose a considerable amount of pounds in no time.

Humus with celery

Calories: 131.2 kcal | Protein: 9.2 grams | Fat: 2.8 grams | Carbohydrates: 17.3 grams Preparation time: 6 minutes Ingredients for one serving: 80 grams of canned chickpeas | 2 cloves of garlic | 2 tbsp cottage cheese | 1 chilli pepper | 2 tbsp orange juice with no added sugar | Salt and pepper | 2 stalks of celery

Preparation:

1. Strain the chickpeas and put them in the blender along with the garlic, cottage cheese, chilli and orange juice.

2. Process into a creamy paste and season with salt and pepper.
3. Cut the celery into pieces and dip the humus with it.
4. This spread also tastes great on a slice of protein bread.
5. You can always prepare the humus anew with different herbs of your choice and different spices.
6. Humus is very healthy and a great source of vitamins and minerals.
7. You should attach great importance to this, especially during a diet.

Small low carb eggplant pizza

Calories: 97.8 kcal | Protein: 8.3 grams | Fat: 5.8 grams | Carbohydrates: 3.1 grams Preparation time: 12 minutes Ingredients for one serving: 4 slices of eggplant approx. 1 cm thick | 3 tbsp pizza tomatoes with no added sugar | 20 grams of Gouda | Oregano | Salt and pepper | 2 tablespoons of canned tuna - in its own juice

Preparation:

1. Briefly sear the aubergines in a grill pan without oil on both sides.

2. Remove from pan and place on a baking sheet lined with baking paper.
3. Salt and pepper and brush with the pizza tomatoes.
4. Sprinkle with Gouda cheese and season with oregano, salt and pepper.
5. Cover with tuna and bake at 200 ° Celsius for 6 minutes on top and bottom heat.
6. You can of course fill the small pizzas as you wish.
7. Whether purely vegetarian or with ham and bacon, there are no limits to the imagination.

Baked zucchini sticks

Calories: 185.8 kcal | Protein: 11.6 grams | Fat: 14.6 grams | Carbohydrates: 2 grams Preparation time: 7 minutes Ingredients for one serving: 1/2 zucchini | 1 egg | 2 tbsp almond flour | 2 tbsp yogurt | Salt and pepper | Oil for deep-frying

Preparation:

1. Cut the zucchini into sticks, season with salt and pepper.

2. Whisk the egg with the almond flour and yoghurt.

3. Pull the sticks through and bake in hot oil.

4. You can also prepare the sticks in the air fryer.

5. Also in the oven with convection and 200! Celsius, the sticks can be baked in about 8 minutes.

6. Enjoy the sticks as a snack or as a side dish, they are a great alternative to traditional French fries.

Carrot cakes

Calories: 141.8 kcal | Protein: 12.6 grams | Fat: 7.4 grams | Carbohydrates: 6.2 grams Preparation time: 8 minutes Ingredients for one serving: 1/2 carrot | 1 egg | 2 tbsp almond flour | Salt and pepper | grated some nutmeg

Preparation:

1. Beat the egg until frothy and finely grate the carrot.

2. Mix the almond flour with the egg and stir in the grated carrot.

3. Season with salt, pepper and nutmeg and bake small pancakes in a non-stick pan.

4. The cakes are a great accompaniment to all dishes with sauces.

5. You can also enjoy this pure or spread it with a little sour cream.

Honey ham omelette

Calories: 225.2 kcal | Protein: 17.9 grams | Fat: 16.4 grams | Carbohydrates: 1.5 grams Preparation time: 6 minutes Ingredients for one serving: 60 grams of honey ham (1 slice) | 1 egg | some thyme | 2 tbsp milk | 1 tbsp chives in rolls | salt and pepper

Preparation:

1. Whisk the egg with the thyme, milk and chives and season with salt and pepper.
2. Pull the ham through and fry in a coated pan.
3. Pour the remaining egg over it.
4. Let stand and turn carefully.
5. If you want, you can add some grated cheese to the egg.

Low carb carrot cheesy fries

Calories: 115 kcal | Protein: 6.4 grams | Fat: 7.8 grams | Carbohydrates: 4.8 grams Preparation time: 15 minutes Ingredients for one serving: 1 carrot | 1 tbsp olive oil | Salt and pepper | 20 grams of grated cheese

Preparation:

1. Cut the carrot into sticks about 0.5 cm thick and place on a baking sheet lined with baking paper.
2. Drizzle with the olive oil and sparingly season with salt and pepper.
3. Heat the tube to 170 ° Celsius and bake the fries on top and bottom heat for 8 minutes.

4. Now sprinkle with the cheese and bake for another 5 minutes.

5. You can also sprinkle the cheesy fries with any herbs of your choice, chilli or cayenne pepper.

Baked peppers with camembert

Calories: 132.5 kcal | Protein: 12.7 grams | Fat: 6.5 grams | Carbohydrates: 5.8 grams Preparation time: 7 minutes Ingredients for one serving: 1/2 yellow pepper | 1/2 red pepper | 30 grams of blackberries | 50 grams of camembert | Freshly ground pepper

Preparation:

1. Cut the peppers into 2 cm thick strips.
2. Line a baking sheet with parchment paper and spread the peppers on top.
3. Top with the blackberries and cover with the sliced camembert.
4. Heat the tube to 200 ° Celsius and bake the peppers on top and bottom heat for about 4 to 5 minutes.
5. This fruity, savory snack is also a great accompaniment to steak and game.

Baked green asparagus with chilli and strawberry dip

Calories: 196.8 kcal | Protein: 13.5 grams | Fat: 14 grams | Carbohydrates: 4.2 grams Preparation time: 10 minutes Ingredients for one serving: 4 stalks of green asparagus | 1 tbsp almond flour | 1 egg | 2 tbsp almonds grated | Salt and pepper | 3 strawberries | 1 tbsp quark

Preparation:

1. Cut off the lower ends of the asparagus and cut in half lengthways.

2. Roll the asparagus in the almond flour.
3. Whisk the egg with salt and pepper and stir in the asparagus.
4. Bread in the almonds and place on a baking sheet lined with baking paper.
5. Bake at 160 ° Celsius and top and bottom heat for 6 minutes.
6. You can also deep-fry the asparagus in the Airfryer.
7. Mash the strawberries with a fork or a magic wand, mix with the quark and sprinkle with a little pepper.
8. Serve the dip with the asparagus.

Pancakes with bacon and cream cheese

Calories: 274.1 kcal | Protein: 24.5 grams | Fat: 17.7 grams | Carbohydrates: 4.2 grams Preparation time: 10 minutes Ingredients for one serving: 2 eggs | 50 ml low-fat milk | 2 tbsp almond flour | Salt and pepper | 1 tbsp parsley chopped | 2 tbsp cream cheese | 2 tbsp bacon diced,

Preparation:

1. Whisk the eggs with the milk and stir with the almond flour until smooth.

2. Season with salt and pepper and stir in the parsley.

3. Process the dough in a coated pan without oil into thin pancakes, so-called pancakes.

4. Remove from the pan, spread the cream cheese and top with the bacon.

5. Beat the pancakes and place on a baking sheet.

6. Bake at 180 ° Celsius for 3 minutes with top and bottom heat.

7. You can briefly toast the bacon in advance in a coated pan.

8. This will make the pancakes extra crispy.

Low carb desserts

Even if you eat the low carb method, that doesn't mean you have to go without sweets. With these tempting recipes you can safely access without regrets and feast to your heart's content.

Baked low carb ice cream in a meringue coating

Calories: 178.4 kcal | Protein: 5.5 grams | Fat: 4.8 grams | Carbohydrates: 28.3 grams Preparation time: 8 minutes Ingredients for one serving: 1 nectarine | 2 small scoops of low carb vanilla ice cream | 1 egg white | 1 tbsp xylitol or sweetener

Preparation:

1. Halve the nectarine and remove the stone.
2. Place a scoop of ice cream in each of the troughs.
3. Beat the egg white with the sweetener to a stiff snow and coat the nectarine and ice with it.
4. Place on a baking sheet lined with baking paper and heat the oven to 220 ° Celsius.
5. Bake the dessert on top and bottom heat for 3 minutes, remove from the oven and enjoy immediately.

Low carb frozen yogurt

Calories: 236.2 kcal | Protein: 11.2 grams | Fat: 14.2 grams | Carbohydrates: 15.9 grams Preparation time: 8 minutes Freezing time: 6 hours Ingredients for one serving: 120 grams of yoghurt | 1 egg white | 1 tbsp xylitol or sweetener | Pulp of half a vanilla pod | some abrasion of an untreated organic lime | 50 ml of cream

Preparation:

1. Mix the yogurt with the egg white, sweetener, vanilla and zest until smooth.
2. Whip the cream until stiff and fold in.
3. Pour the mixture into a bowl and freeze for at least 6 hours.
4. Remove from the freezer and use the blender to make a frozen yoghurt.
5. Serve with fresh berries as required and enjoy.

Berries au gratin

Calories: 117.5 kcal | Protein: 5.9 grams | Fat: 4.7 grams | Carbohydrates: 12.9 grams Preparation time: 10 minutes Ingredients for one serving: 80 grams of fresh or frozen berry mix | 1 egg | Juice and zest of half an untreated organic orange | 1 teaspoon xylitol, stevia or sweetener as required

Preparation:

1. Beat the egg with the orange juice and the sweetener over a hot water bath until frothy.
2. Put the berries in a small baking dish and marinate with the zest.
3. Pour the egg mixture over them.
4. Heat the oven to 220 ° Celsius and grill the berries for 4 minutes on top and bottom heat.
5. You can also enjoy the gratinated berries with a scoop of low-carb ice cream.

Apple crumble with low carb streusel

Calories: 273.4 kcal | Protein: 11.2 grams | Fat: 20.2 grams | Carbohydrates: 11.7 grams Preparation time: 12 minutes Ingredients for one serving: 1/2 apple | 1 squirt of lemon juice | 20 grams of butter | 30 grams of almond flour | 1 pinch of cinnamon | some abrasion of an untreated organic orange | Sweetener as needed

Preparation:

1. Cut the apple into thin wedges and layer in a small tart pan.
2. Drizzle with the lemon juice.
3. Melt the butter in a pan and stir in the almond flour along with the cinnamon and the sweetener.
4. Stir until the mixture loosens crumbly from the bottom of the pan.
5. Now distribute these crumbs over the apples, flavor with the zest and put in the oven.
6. Bake at 180 ° Celsius for 10 minutes with top and bottom heat.

Seductive low carb brownies

Calories: 2972.3 kcal | Protein: 47.5 grams | Fat: 187.5 grams | Carbohydrates: 273.7 grams Preparation time: 25 minutes Ingredients for approx. 12 brownies: 120 grams of butter | 3 eggs | 250 grams of dark chocolate xylitol | 80 grams of xylitol or stevia as required | 60 grams of almond flour | 2 tbsp double-defoiled cocoa | 1 pack of baking powder | 1 pinch of Himalayan rock salt

Preparation:

1. Beat the butter until frothy and stir one egg at a time into the butter.

2. Melt the chocolate in a small pan, stirring constantly, and stir quickly into the butter mixture.

3. Stir in the sweetener, almond flour, cocoa, baking powder and salt.

4. Pour the dough into a lightly buttered baking dish.

5. The dimensions 25 cm x 25 cm fit this perfectly.

6. Heat the oven to 175 ° Celsius and bake the brownies on top and bottom heat for 20 minutes.

7. Take out of the oven and cut into 12 pieces.

8. The nutritional information in this recipe is based on 12 pieces.

Low carb muffins with ginger and vanilla

Calories: 943.1 kcal | Protein: 43.3 grams | Fat: 81.1 grams | Carbohydrates: 10 grams Preparation time: 20 minutes Ingredients for 4 muffins: 2 eggs | 90 grams of almond flour | 1 pack of baking powder | 3 tbsp Greek yogurt | Pulp of a vanilla pod or vanilla flavor | 1 pinch of freshly grated ginger or powder | 2 tbsp chopped walnuts | 4 walnut halves

Preparation:

1. Separate the eggs and use the whisk or hand mixer to work the egg white into a stiff snow.

2. Mix the egg yolks with the Greek yogurt until smooth and work in the almond flour and baking powder.

3. Stir in vanilla, ginger and chopped walnuts and then carefully fold in the egg whites.

4. Fill the batter into four muffin tins.

5. Place one walnut half on each muffin.

6. Heat the oven to 170 ° Celsius and bake the muffins on top and bottom heat for about 15 minutes.

7. You can serve the muffins with a top made of whipped vanilla cream and you can conjure up low carb cup cakes in no time at all.

Low carb chocolate ice cream

Calories: 1130.2 kcal | Protein: 26.3 grams | Fat: 66.6 grams | Carbohydrates: 106.4 grams Preparation time: 10 minutes Freezing time: at least 6 hours Ingredients for four servings: 2 eggs | 1 egg white | 100 grams of dark chocolate xylitol | 2 tbsp xylitol, stevia or sweetener | 200 ml of cream

Preparation:

1. Beat the eggs with the sweetener until frothy and stir in the egg white.

2. Melt the chocolate over a hot water bath.

3. Quickly stir into the egg mixture with the whisk.

4. Whip the cream until stiff and fold in carefully.

5. Pour the mass into a tub and freeze for at least 6 hours.

6. Remove from the freezer and take out a total of 4 servings of ice.

7. The nutritional information is calculated for 4 whole servings.

Crepes with berry sauce

Calories: 418.6 kcal | Protein: 17.1 grams | Fat: 33.4 grams | Carbohydrates: 12.4 grams Preparation time: 9 minutes Ingredients for one serving: 2 egg yolks | 60 ml cream | 2 tbsp coconut flour | 1 pinch of Himalayan salt | 50 grams of wild berries fresh or frozen | 2 tbsp cottage cheese | 1 teaspoon xylitol or sweetener | some abrasion of an untreated organic orange

Preparation:

1. Whisk the egg yolks with the cream and stir with the coconut flour and salt until smooth.
2. In a non-stick pan, bake the dough into thin crepes without fat.
3. Puree the berries with the cottage cheese, sweetener and zest with the magic wand.
4. Pour the sauce over the crepes and serve.
5. Sprinkle with a little powder xylitol as needed.
6. Even a dollop of cream goes perfectly with this small, fruity delicacy.

Yogurt pudding with jelly

Calories: 163.6 kcal | Protein: 12.4 grams | Fat: 6.8 grams | Carbohydrates: 13.2 grams Preparation time: 8 minutes Cooling time: at least 4 hours Ingredients for one serving: 150 grams of yoghurt | 1 tsp chia seeds | 1 tbsp xylitol or sweetener | some vanilla flavor | some abrasion of an untreated organic lime | 50 ml freshly squeezed grapefruit juice | 1 pinch of instant gelatine

Preparation:

1. Mix the yogurt with the chia seeds, the sweetener, the vanilla and the lime zest until smooth.
2. Pour into a glass.
3. Mix the grapefruit juice well with the instant gelatine until it has completely dissolved.
4. Spread over the yoghurt and let set in the refrigerator for at least 4 hours, preferably overnight.

Low carb carrot muffins with cinnamon and cocoa

Calories: 964.4 kcal | Protein: 49.8 grams | Fat: 77.6 grams | Carbohydrates: 16.7 grams Preparation time: 20 minutes Ingredients for 4 muffins: 60 grams of butter | 2 eggs | 2 tbsp yogurt | 90 grams of almond flour | 1/2 pack of baking powder | 100 grams of carrots finely grated | 2 tbsp finely chopped pistachios | 1 pinch of cinnamon | 1 tbsp double-defoiled cocoa | 1 pinch of Himalayan salt | 2 dashes of sweetener

Preparation:

1. Beat the butter until frothy and stir one egg at a time into the butter.

2. Mix with the almond flour and incorporate baking powder, yogurt, carrots, pistachios, cinnamon, cocoa, salt and sweetener.

3. Divide the mixture into four muffin tins. Bake at 180 ° Celsius with top and bottom heat for 15 minutes.